## The Natural Way Series

Increasing numbers of people worldwide are falling victim to illnesses which modern medicine, for all its technical advances, seems often powerless to prevent – and sometimes actually causes. To help with these so-called 'diseases of civilization' more and more people are turning to 'natural' medicine for an answer. *The Natural Way* series aims to offer clear, practical and reliable guidance to the safest, gentlest and most effective treatments available – and so to give sufferers and their families the information they need to make their own choices about the most suitable treatments.

**Special note from the Publisher**

A variety of terms such as 'alternative medicine', 'complementary medicine', 'holistic medicine' and 'unorthodox medicine' are commonly used to describe many of the treatments mentioned in this book – but because in practice they all mean much the same the publishers have opted for the single term 'natural' to cover them all. 'Natural' in the context of this series means treatments which are first and foremost gentle, safe and effective, and avoid the use of toxic drugs or surgery. The treatments described are mostly tried and tested, and many have been proven to be effective in medical trials, but some have not. Where treatments are interesting and intriguing but speculative at present, this has been clearly indicated.

**The books in this series are intended for information and guidance only. They are not intended to replace professional advice, and readers are strongly urged to consult an experienced practitioner for a proper diagnosis or assessment before trying any of the treatments outlined.**

*Other titles in* The Natural Way *series*

Arthritis & Rheumatism
Asthma
Back Pain
Cancer
Colds & Flu
Diabetes
Eczema
Heart Disease
HIV & Aids
Infertility
Irritable Bowel Syndrome
Migraine
Multiple Sclerosis
Premenstrual Syndrome
Psoriasis

# THE NATURAL WAY

# Cystitis

*Jacqueline Young*

*Series medical consultants*
*Dr Peter Albright MD (USA)*
*& Dr David Peters MD (UK)*

Approved by the
AMERICAN HOLISTIC MEDICAL ASSOCIATION
& BRITISH HOLISTIC MEDICAL ASSOCIATION

ELEMENT
Shaftesbury, Dorset • Rockport, Massachusetts
Brisbane, Queensland

for Jacaranda Wiley Limited
33 Park Road, Milton, Brisbane 4064



Cover design by Max Fairbrother
Text illustrations by David Gifford
Designed and typeset by Linda Reed and Joss Nizan
Printed and bound in Great Britain by
Biddles Limited, Guildford and King's Lynn

British Library Cataloguing in Publication
data available

Library of Congress Cataloging in Publication
data available

ISBN 1-85230-889-3

# Contents


| | | |
|---|---|---|
| *List of illustrations* | | vi |
| *Acknowledgements* | | viii |
| *Introduction* | | ix |
| Chapter 1 | **What is cystitis?** | 1 |
| Chapter 2 | **All about the urinary system** | 5 |
| Chapter 3 | **Common causes of cystitis** | 11 |
| Chapter 4 | **Self-help for cystitis** | 21 |
| Chapter 5 | **Conventional treatments and procedures** | 37 |
| Chapter 6 | **Natural therapies and cystitis** | 44 |
| Chapter 7 | **Treating the body** | 53 |
| Chapter 8 | **Treating the mind** | 90 |
| Chapter 9 | **Diet and nutrition** | 100 |
| Chapter 10 | **How to find and choose a natural therapist** | 103 |
| *Appendix A* | **Useful organizations** | 111 |
| *Appendix B* | **Useful further reading** | 115 |
| *Index* | | 117 |

## Illustrations

*Figure 1* *Male and female urinary systems* 7
*Figure 2* *Forward bending pose* 25
*Figure 3* *Acupressure points for cystitis* 59
*Figure 4* *Reflex points for the urinary system* 89

This book is dedicated to

**Angela Kilmartin**

who has done more than anyone
to increase public and medical
awareness of cystitis
and show how to prevent it

## Acknowledgements

Thank are due to all those who have shared their experience of cystitis and to the practitioners who have shared their expertise and case histories. They include Richard Blackwell BMedSci, MBAcC; Joe Goodman, ND, DO, DrAc; Professor Laurie Hartman, DO, MRO, PhD; Clare Harvey, DipShenTao, MIFVM; Dr Connie Hernandez, ND; Dr Richard James, MB, BS, LicAc, MBAcC, MBMAS, DipHumPsych; Dr Julian Kenyon, MD, MB, ChB; Dr Patrick Kingsley, MB, BS, MRCS, LRCP, FAAEM, DA, DObst, RCOG; Jane Lethem, MPsychol; Naresh Maini, BPharm, MRPharmS; Felicity Moir, DipHerb, MBAcC; Deirdre St John, DO, MRO; Gretchen de Soriano, MRCHM, MKANPO, MBAcC, DipMCCA; and Roger Newman Turner, BAc, ND, DO.

Thanks also to Alison Gould, of the Acupuncture Research Resource Centre; Peter Deadman, editor of the *Journal of Chinese Medicine*; Rohit Mehta and Gareth Cork at the Nutri Centre, London; Martin Powell at East West Herbs; Caroline Guy and Samantha Christie of Lamberts Healthcare Ltd, and Sandra McDade for providing references and product information; to Dr Andrew Lockie and Penguin Books and Dr Patrick Kingsley and Ebury Press for permission to quote from their books; to Angela Kilmartin and Thorsons/HarperCollins for permission to reproduce her bottle washing technique, and to Angela herself for her comments and seemingly limitless enthusiasm on the subject of the prevention of cystitis; to Chris McLaughlin and Sheila Brown for typing assistance; to the series editor Richard Thomas and Julia McCutchen at Element Books for their patience and support; and lastly to my precious and delightful young son, Michael, who put up with all the hours mummy spent on the computer and kept me laughing in between, and to his 'minders', especially my mother, Joanne Angel, Don Angel, Angela, Elena, Emma and Louise.

# Introduction

Cystitis is a bladder condition that afflicts millions of adults and children worldwide every year. Its symptoms of burning sensations when passing urine, abdominal pain, and fever are incapacitating and distressing. Cystitis frequently recurs and can have a devastating effect on a person's life. It can also be dangerous, and even life-threatening, if the infection is untreated and allowed to spread up to the kidneys.

Yet cystitis is largely preventable if good hygiene practices are followed and certain changes in diet and lifestyle are implemented. There really is no need for this appalling suffering and the main barrier to preventing it is simply ignorance. There is ignorance among adults and children themselves about preventive techniques and, sadly, ignorance among many members of the medical profession about recognizing the true causes of cystitis and the best ways to prevent it.

Cystitis is an unglamorous subject and the medical profession was initially slow to recognize the different types of cystitis and their causes. Antibiotic treatment used to be prescribed routinely and this often led to a cycle of thrush and re-infection. More recently pioneers from both within and outside the profession have drawn attention to cystitis and clarified the distinction between bacterial and non-bacterial cystitis and the role of other factors such as *candida* and food intolerances.

This means there is no excuse for ignorance any longer and it is up to every health practitioner and, indeed, every adult to inform themselves about cystitis and to pass on what they know to children so that their lives need not be blighted either.

Further advances also need to be made in understanding why some people get cystitis and others do not. It is not enough to simply put cystitis down to invading bacteria or irritated tissues. We need to look at why the person's immune system and powers of resistance have been unable to deal with and expel the bacteria or why their tissues have become irritated and unable to heal. Maybe their general health and vitality is poor, their diet inadequate and their lifestyle over-demanding. There could also be some organic imbalance which is predisposing them to cystitis. Assessing them and treating them as whole people, rather than merely treating a bladder condition, will increase the likelihood of promoting both healing and general health improvement.

The natural therapies may help us approach cystitis in this way. To date they have been largely ignored, or given only a cursory role in the treatment of cystitis yet they have a tremendous amount to offer in terms of both the treatment of cystitis and the self-help techniques which can prevent it. Herbal and homoeopathic treatments can help boost immunity and ease bladder irritation, acupuncture can improve urinary function and structural therapies may improve circulation to and from the pelvic organs. Natural therapies enable the emotional and mental aspects of cystitis to be addressed too. All too often there are fears and anxieties which play a part in its development.

The standards of training in natural therapies and public awareness of the therapies are increasing all the time. There is also a growing body of research into the efficacy of these therapies and increasing co-operation between their practitioners and the medical profession.

It's to be hoped that this will lead to a more integrated approach to health and disease that utilizes the best of all medical systems.

I myself suffered recurrent cystitis from the time I was a teenager to my early 20's. At that time I discovered Angela Kilmartin's pioneering book, *Understanding Cystitis* and it literally changed my life, virtually putting an end to the misery of cystitis overnight. Over the next two decades, training and practising in orthodox and complementary medical approaches, I have maintained a special interest in cystitis and how to prevent it. This research and clinical experience has enabled me to help countless individuals, including myself, to put a stop to cystitis once and for all. It is a joy to have the opportunity, in this book, to share what I have learnt and found to be effective for the benefit of others.

The central aim of this book is to suggest that a careful combination of tried and tested self-help techniques, orthodox medical approaches and natural therapies is the best way to deal with cystitis. I believe such an approach can enable us to eradicate cystitis forever and build general health, vitality and wellbeing at the same time.

Jacqueline Young
Hertfordshire, England.
August 1996

CHAPTER 1

# What is cystitis?

## *How and why cystitis develops and whom it affects*

Cystitis is an inflammation of the bladder caused by infection by invading bacteria or by irritation of the delicate tissues lining the bladder and the urinary passages. It is one of the commonest disorders of the urinary system and one of the most frequent complaints presented at doctors' surgeries. It represents millions of consultations per year worldwide and is thought to be a major cause of work loss particularly among the female population.

The word cystitis literally means inflammation of the urinary bladder. (*Kystis* refers to the bladder and *itis* means inflammation.) It is characterized by an increased desire to pass urine and a burning sensation when doing so. The sensation may be one of mild irritation and discomfort or it can be excruciatingly painful. At the very least cystitis is uncomfortable and distressing while at worst it can be excruciatingly painful and even dangerous as, untreated, it can lead to serious kidney problems.

Cystitis is most common among adult women but men and children, especially young girls, can be affected too. Many are reluctant to discuss this painful and embarrassing condition, yet it can have a serious effect on their lives, disrupting work and daily schedules, destroying social life, preventing love-making, wrecking relationships and leading to deep fatigue and despair.

## Causes of cystitis

The causes of cystitis are many and diverse. A major cause is bacteria entering the urethra, the tube leading to the bladder, having been passed from the openings of the anus and vagina. The spread of the bacteria may be influenced by the strength of the person's immune system which influences the body's ability to fight and expel the bacteria. Anatomical problems can also play a part. For example, polyps can obstruct the free flow of urine and fissures (tears) in the lining of the urethral and bladder walls can provide an ideal site for the bacteria to breed.

Other non-bacterial factors such as diet, lifestyle, and allergies need to be considered too. They can be triggers leading to inflammation of the tissues lining the urethra and bladder. As acidic urine comes into contact with the inflamed tissue the result is pain.

These causes will be discussed in detail in Chapter 3.

## Symptoms of cystitis

Symptoms vary according to the individual but most people will experience some or all of the following symtoms.

- **A burning sensation on passing urine.** This can range from mild discomfort to agonizing pain.
- **An increased desire to pass urine.** Typically you keep feeling the need to go to the toilet yet are only able to pass a few, painful drops of urine when you do go. When symptoms are really bad you may feel unable to leave the toilet at all. You can end up sitting there for long periods through the night clutched in pain and misery.
- **Strong-smelling urine that may contain blood.** As the urine becomes more concentrated its odour increases

noticeably. Blood in the urine is a serious symptom that must be medically investigated.

- **Pain in the abdomen and lower back.** Aching or stabbing pain may be felt in the area of the bladder, around the lower abdomen, or in the area of the kidneys (just below the waist in the lower back) as these organs become affected.
- **Alternating fever and chills.** You may feel hot one moment, especially in the face and upper body, and chilly throughout the body the next. Fever is felt particularly when the inflammation is severe, while chills may be a sign that the kidneys are becoming affected.
- **Exhaustion and anxiety.** The pain and discomfort of cystitis is tiring and anxiety-provoking. You may ache all over, feel nauseous and develop a headache to add to your existing symptoms. Psychologically you can begin to feel hopeless and despairing.

Symptoms are often worse at night, particularly if you reduce your intake of fluids and your urine becomes more concentrated. The symptoms are usually mild at first and then increase in severity as the cystitis develops. This is one reason why preventive action should be taken as soon as symptoms appear (*see* page 31).

### Who is affected?

Anyone can be affected by cystitis. Women in their 20s, 30s and 40s, especially those that are sexually active, are most vulnerable. (Epidemiological studies have shown that nuns are one-tenth as likely to get cystitis as married women.) However, elderly women, especially those suffering from incontinence (inability to control the flow of urine) or poor mobility leading to poor hygiene, are also commonly affected. Various surveys have suggested that around one in three of all women, and three times as many women as men, will be affected by cystitis at some time in their lives.

Men are affected less often than women mainly because of differences in male anatomy (*see* page 7). Men can suffer from urethral inflammation, known as non-specific urethritis (NSU), but in many cases their urinary problems are due to prostate gland enlargement or infection rather than bladder infection.

Children may also develop cystitis, but again females are far more likely to be affected than males. One American report states that only 0.05 per cent of young boys develop urinary tract infections but for young girls it rises to two to five per cent. Female babies can develop urinary infections too and this may be due to poor baby hygiene by the parents as much as to the baby's anatomy.

The numbers of people affected may be even higher than we think as several studies have revealed an under-reporting of symptoms. In one study of 5,000 school children randomly selected from a sample of 100,000, a third were found to have cystitis-type symptoms and 13 per cent had evidence of urinary tract infection although they had not presented these symptoms to their family doctors. This means that the scale of the problem and the amount of suffering caused by cystitis is enormous.

CHAPTER 2

# All about the urinary system

*The parts of the body affected by cystitis*

Urine, a waste product of the body, is made in the kidneys and then passed down to the bladder via two tubes, the ureters, one from each kidney. The bladder is a hollow bag, located in the pelvis, which temporarily stores the urine until it is ready to be passed out of the body. In women the bladder lies in front of the womb, or uterus, while in men it is located in front of the lower end of the large intestine, the rectum.

When the bladder is empty it is approximately the size of a fist and its shape is triangular. As it fills with urine it expands like a ball in the lower abdomen. The bladder receives urine from the kidneys in a steady dribble that continues 24 hours a day. As the urine enters the bladder via the ureters, valves at the end of each tube seal the urine in the bladder and prevent it going back up to the kidneys.

The two kidneys are located at the back of the body on either side of the spine just below the lower ribs. They are about 10 centimetres long and 6 centimetres wide and weigh about 5 ounces (140gm) each. Together they act as important filters for the blood, removing waste products and regulating the levels of sodium, potassium and calcium. The kidneys filter approximately two pints of liquid every minute and about one per cent of this fluid is discharged in the form of urine made up of waste products, mainly in the form of urea, and excess water.

Our bodies are 70 per cent water and every day we lose large amounts through sweat, through urination and via the air that we exhale, so we constantly need to take in new fluid. Almost half of what we drink every day is passed out of the body as urine.

## The bladder

As the bladder fills with urine the muscles in the bladder wall are stretched, the pressure inside the bladder rises and causes a desire to urinate. In most people the bladder can comfortably store up to half a pint of liquid before they feel the urge to pass urine, but if the amount increases to a pint, or more, increasing discomfort is felt.

In babies, the emptying of the bladder is automatic and uncontrolled but in adults the mechanism is controlled via the nervous system. This allows us to tolerate some distension and discomfort until we can conveniently empty the bladder.

As the amount of liquid in the bladder increases, the muscles in the bladder wall start to contract. When they reach their maximum contraction urine is expelled from the bladder via a tube called the urethra. The flow of urine down this tube is controlled by two valves, one at the top of the tube, that seals urine in the bladder until it is ready to be expelled, and one at the lower end of the tube.

### *How bladder infection occurs*

For bladder infection to occur bacteria must pass up the urethra and enter the bladder.

In men the urethra is 18 to 20 centimetres long and passes via the prostate gland along the length of the penis to the exterior. It is therefore quite difficult for

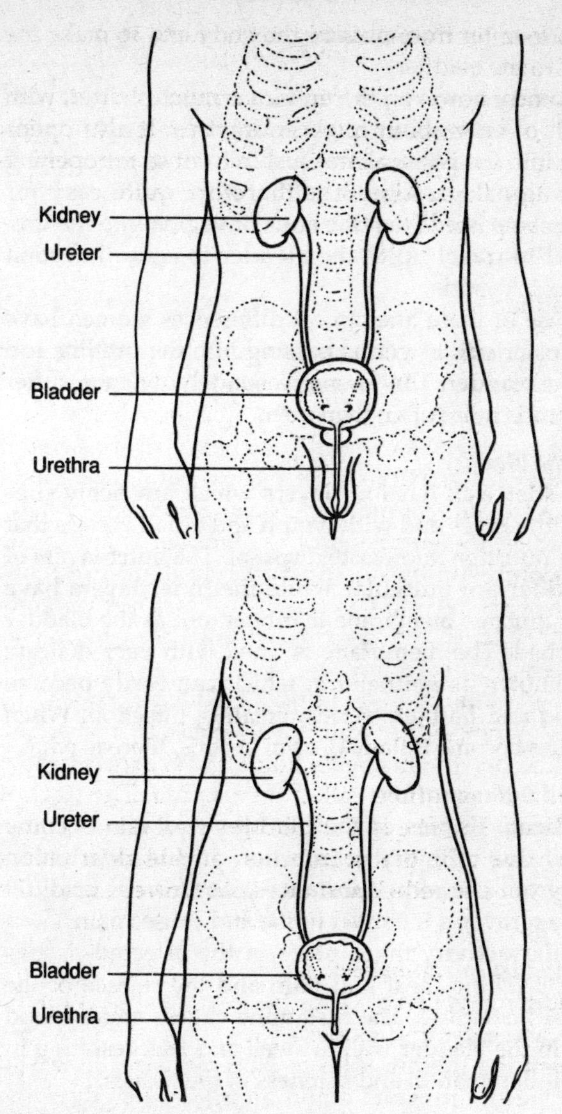


**Fig. 1 Male and female urinary systems**

bacteria to enter from outside the body and to make the journey to the bladder.

In women, however, the urethra is much shorter, with a length of only about four centimetres. It also opens directly into the perineal area just in front of the opening of the vaginal passage. It is therefore quite easy for germs to be passed from the anus or vagina into the urethra and to travel up to the bladder to cause infection resulting in cystitis.

Because of these anatomical differences women have a far greater risk of germs passing into the urethra and up to the bladder. This is one reason why women suffer from cystitis more often than men.

### *Inside the bladder*

The bladder wall has four layers which are richly supplied with nerves and with lymph and blood vessels that provide nutrition and waste disposal. The outer layers of the bladder are muscular while the inner layers have folds of mucous membrane that open out as the bladder is stretched. The membrane is lined with very delicate tissue, known as epithelium, which can easily become damaged and harbour germs, creating infection. When the tissues become inflamed, as in cystitis, there is pain.

### *Pain and inflammation*

The delicate tissues of the bladder wall can become inflamed due to injury or infection or due to irritation caused from chemical substances. As urine is acidic it further aggravates inflamed tissue and causes pain.

Cellular activity takes place in the affected tissues causing swelling, heat and pain and the release of the chemical histamine. The histamine causes small blood vessels in the bladder wall to swell and leak resulting in further inflammation and soreness in the tissues.

As the leaked fluid in the tissues accumulates and the nerve endings become irritated, increasing pain is felt. In cystitis the pain is most commonly felt in the urethra and at the base of the bladder.

***Scarring and re-infection***

As the body deals with cystitis, white blood cells help to destroy any bacteria causing infection, dead tissue cells are broken down and removed and new tissue is formed. However, scar tissue can remain, with small cracks that can easily break open and bleed again. This makes re-infection and re-inflammation more likely in the future and is one reason why cystitis may occur with increasing frequency and severity.

## Diagnosing cystitis

The first stage of diagnosis is on the basis of symptoms, that is, increased frequency of urination, burning pain on passing water, fever and chills and so on. However, clinically, it is vital that urine samples are taken and analysed to establish exactly which, if any, bacteria are present and to determine the best course of treatment to eradicate any infection.

Your family doctor will almost always ask for a urine sample. You can either provide it at the surgery or take it at home at the first sign of infection and deliver it to the surgery as quickly as possible to be sent for analysis. Care must be taken to take the sample correctly and to avoid contamination (*see* Urine Samples and Urine Testing, pages 37–38). If bacteria are found in the urine sample further tests will be done overnight to establish which drug will be most effective in eradicating the infection (*see* pages 39–40) and this will then be prescribed.

## Differentiating between cystitis and other genito-urinary infections

To differentiate between urethral, bladder and vaginal infections, samples of both initial and mid-stream urine may be taken as well as vaginal swabs so that the levels of bacteria can be compared. Additional internal examinations, investigations, scans, etc may also be taken to check the position of the internal organs, check they are functioning correctly and test for the presence of any other abnormalities, such as tumours (*see* page 42–43).

## Risk factors and the development of cystitis into other conditions

If untreated, or treated incorrectly, bladder infection can spread to the kidneys and can seriously damage them. The damage may be irreversible and can even be fatal. Inflammation of the kidneys (nephritis) may be characterized by scanty, blood-stained urine and pronounced puffiness and swelling of the face and limbs (oedema). In more chronic stages there is extensive tissue damage in the kidneys which can lead to kidney failure. To prevent the risk of kidney infection it is vital that cystitis is accurately diagnosed and properly treated.

CHAPTER 3

# Common causes of cystitis

*The different causes of cystitis and how they affect the body*

The causes of cystitis can broadly be divided into two main groups, those that are due to bacterial infection and those not due to infection. However, in diagnosis this distinction can be blurred by two factors.

First, many cases diagnosed as non-bacterial may actually have a bacterial cause that remains undetected because of errors in the urine sampling procedure. If the person drinks before taking the sample and dilutes it, or if the sample is taken late in the day or not stored correctly, test results may be negative even though bacteria are present.

On the other hand, a urine test may be positive, but the original cause of the infection may be lowered immunity and resistance, as a result of underlying dietary or lifestyle factors, rather than the mere presence of the bacteria. Bacteria enter the body all the time but the body's ability to recognize, fight and expel the bacteria is crucial. When this resistance mechanism fails the bacteria can take hold and infection will result.

**Bacterial cystitis**

In bacterial cystitis, invading bacteria enter the urethra and pass up to the bladder to spread infection. The bacteria generally responsible are *Escherichia coli (E. coli)* which is commonly found in the anus and in faeces. These bacteria may be able to enter the urethra due to:

- incorrect wiping after going to the toilet
- poor hygiene of the genital region
- sexual positions or practices
- incorrect use of tampons (not changed regularly and/or used too much of the time)

Lifestyle factors such as type of clothing, posture, and the presence of irritants such as strong soaps or perfumes can aggravate the problem (*see* section below).

It is essential to have urine tests performed in order to determine the presence of this bacterium. If it is found then prompt treatment, usually in the form of antibiotics (*see* Chapter 5), is essential in order to prevent the spread of infection, via the ureters, to the kidneys.

### Non-bacterial cystitis

Non-bacterial cystitis is where the symptoms of cystitis are evident but there are no detectable bacteria present. In this case the cause of the symptoms is inflammation of the delicate epithelial tissue in the bladder or the lining of the urethra due to one or more of the following:

- exposure to chemical irritants such as strongly perfumed soaps, deodorants or heavily chlorinated swimming pools
- food irritants and/or allergies, such as additives, flavourings, an excess of highly spiced or acidic foods
- inadequate intake of fluids leading to dehydration and increased concentration of the urine, or excess intake of fluids that irritate the bladder such as coffee, tea, alcohol, fruit juices and colas

- reaction to certain forms of contraception such as the pill, spermicidal creams or the plastic used in caps and diaphragms
- foreign bodies such as dirt or sand introduced to the urethra due to poor hygiene or certain sexual practices
- exposure of the perineal area to extreme hot or cold, for example sitting on radiators or cold floors or remaining in wet, cold swimming costumes for long periods
- vibration and friction due to movement when travelling or horse riding

This type of cystitis is sometimes labelled 'interstitial cystitis' but it should be noted that the frequency of this diagnosis varies enormously from area to area and country to country. For example, such a diagnosis is far more common in the USA than in the UK and is more common in certain parts of the north of England than in the south. The high discrepancy has led some people to argue that 'interstitial cystitis' is a label that depends on the diagnostic style of certain doctors and surgeons rather than it being a reality. In some cases originally diagnosed as interstitial cystitis bacteria were in fact found when urine samples were repeated and taken correctly.

## Causative factors

Each of the causative factors will now be examined in detail. Recognizing them and changing them is the key to self-help and the prevention of cystitis.

### *1 Hygiene*

The most common cause of cystitis is poor hygiene. For women and girls in particular, because of the proximity of the urethral opening with the anus and the vaginal passage, it is very easy for bacteria to be spread and to enter the urethral tube and travel up to the bladder. If the body is not capable of overcoming and expelling the bacteria, infection results. Irritants may also enter the body the same way (see section on irritants below). It is therefore vital to ensure a good hygiene routine that includes wiping from front to back after going to the toilet, regular, gentle cleansing of the perineal area and always passing urine before and after intercourse. All of these measures are discussed in detail in the chapter on self-help (Chapter 4).

Poor hygiene can be the cause of cystitis in young girls and even babies if the parents do not learn how to clean them properly when changing nappies or do not teach good toilet habits as they grow older. In men, too, poor hygiene, especially before and after sex, may result in the spread of bacteria, so regular washing of the hands and penis are essential (*see* Chapter 4).

2 *Sex*

Sex is another major cause of cystitis in both women and men. If the woman is not sufficiently aroused prior to penetration, or if she is going through the menopause and suffering from dryness as a result of falling oestrogen levels, the vaginal passage may not be sufficiently lubricated and bruising can result. Small cuts in the delicate lining of the vaginal passage, or inflammation of the tissues, can provide breeding grounds for unfriendly bacteria that may enter with the penis. As these spread they can easily be passed into the urethra and cystitis can result.

Very active sex or certain love-making positions that involve a lot of friction can also irritate the lining of the vaginal passage or the tip of the penis making the tissues prone to infection.

***3 Vaginal health***

If there is a vaginal infection, such as thrush, the bacteria *E. coli* will be present and may be passed from the vaginal opening across to the urethra. As the *E. coli* spread up the urethra and multiply, bladder infection may result.

***4 Digestion***

If digestion is poor and you suffer from constipation this may also help bring about cystitis. Constipation leads to a build up of toxins in the body and impaired immune function, both of which will lower the body's resistance to infection.

A build-up of faecal matter in the intestinal walls increases pressure in the lower abdomen and can put pressure on the bladder, impairing its function and making it more prone to inflammation or infection.

***5 Position of the bladder or uterus***

The position of the bladder and the uterus in a woman's pelvic cavity varies slightly from person to person. Different positions affect the smooth flow and drainage of blood and lymph (clear fluid carried in the lymph vessels) which can affect susceptibility to, and resistance to, infection. The free flow of urine in the urinary tract can also be affected.

If the neck of the bladder is very tight, or the muscles of the bladder are weak, it may be difficult to empty the bladder fully. Stale urine remaining in the bladder can become a breeding ground for invading bacteria.

Pregnancy, childbirth, hysterectomy and menopause can all affect bladder function and create the conditions for cystitis. For example, weakened pelvic floor muscles increase the likelihood of prolapse of the uterus resulting in incomplete emptying of the bladder and creating an opportunity for bacteria to breed. Scar tissue, such as around episiotomy scars, can contain tiny fissures where bacteria get trapped and then multiply. Hormonal changes can lead to dryness and affect the mucous membranes making infection more likely.

*6 Toilet training*

Children given poor toilet training can be vulnerable to cystitis. The child may not be encouraged to go the toilet regularly or to empty the bladder fully. Young girls in particular may develop the habit of retaining urine and postponing going to the toilet for as long as possible. This habit may continue at school if the child does not like using the school toilets or is forbidden to use them during lessons. The habit can then continue into adulthood.

Retention of urine means increased pressure on the bladder and infrequent flushing out of the urethra which means bacteria are not expelled and infection can develop.

*7 Congenital weakness*

Certain individuals may have a predisposition to urinary infections. This could be because of anatomy, such as the position of the relevant organs in the body, or the length of the urethra, as already mentioned, or the cause may be more 'energetic'. According to Oriental medical theory a person is born with a certain amount of vitality that is inherited from the parents. This vitality is reflected in the strength of the kidney meridians. Acupuncturists argue that if the kidney meridian is weak from birth there may be predisposition to urinary infections (*see* section on acupuncture in Chapter 7).

*8 Contraception*

Certain individuals react badly to the chemicals contained in spermicidal creams, to different types of contraceptive pill, or to the substances used in manufacturing condoms. A recent paper in the *New England Journal of Medicine* reported that among 800 sexually active young women those using spermicidal creams for contraception had a significantly higher chance of developing an infection than those using other methods. The level of risk increased with the frequency of use.

***9 Irritants***

As well as the contraceptives mentioned above, irritants may come in the form of perfumed soaps or bath and shower products and strong chemical washing powders. The irritants can be passed directly into the body in the water surrounding the urethral opening during a bath or shower, or be passed on a flannel. They may also directly enter the body in vaginal douches.

Alternatively, the irritants may enter via the mouth in the form of food additives, colourings or other foods that the person is allergic to. Carried in the blood stream, these substances may irritate tissues weakened by previous infection or scarring. They can also lead to the production of histamine by the body's defence system which can cause the small blood vessels in the bladder wall to swell and leak, leading to inflammation and potential infection.

***10 Diet and liquid intake***

Diet plays a crucial role in the development of cystitis and in the frequency of attacks. All foods have acid or alkaline properties and a highly acidic diet, for example containing lots of red meat, dairy products, sugar and alcohol, all of which are acid-forming in the body, can increase the acidic content of the urine and aggravate the symptoms of cystitis.

The vitamin and mineral balance in the body, especially the balance of sodium and potassium which is regulated by the kidneys, is also important, as is the amount of liquid intake. Adults drinking less than four pints of fluids a day, or consuming large amounts of diuretics such as coffee or alcohol which dehydrate the body, will have more concentrated urine and are more likely to suffer urinary discomfort. Many children also drink insufficient liquids or too many highly sweetened or carbonated drinks which further acidify both blood and urine.

### *11 Posture*

Nowadays many people live quite sedentary lives, seated much of the time, travelling in cars, and with insufficient exercise. As a result muscle tone diminishes, posture deteriorates and the internal organs are poorly supported. Circulation of blood and lymph is also affected and this can play a role in cystitis. When there is congestion in the pelvic region there is poor nourishment of the tissues and low resistance to infection.

### *12 Environment*

Extremes of temperature can help trigger cystitis. Many people suffer from cystitis for the first time when they are abroad in a hot climate and do not drink sufficient fluids to keep the body well hydrated. As a result, the urine becomes increasingly concentrated and discomfort can result. The situation can be worsened if there is a change of diet, increased consumption of alcohol or sexual contact.

Cystitis can also be triggered by prolonged exposure of the pelvic region to hot or cold temperatures. Sitting on a hot radiator in winter may feel comforting but it will cause the sensitive tissues in the genital region to swell and become inflamed. Alternatively, sitting on a cold floor or remaining in a cold, wet swimsuit for long periods can chill the lower regions of the body, weakening resistance to infection and creating disturbance in bladder function.

### *13 Medication*

Cystitis sufferers can become caught in a vicious cycle of attack, medication and re-infection. If the cystitis is bacterial it is common to take antibiotics in order to eradicate the infection and prevent it spreading to the kidneys. The antibiotics can eradicate the infection but they do not help repair tissue damage. Also, repeated use of antibiotics can disturb the delicate balance of micro-organisms in the large intestine and the vagina and a proliferation of the micro-organism, *candida* or thrush, a yeast infection, can result. This can compound the misery of the cystitis sufferer and also increase the likelihood of a recurrence.

### *14 Stress*

Lastly, stress plays a significant role in cystitis. Many people have very demanding daily schedules, often working long hours and maybe juggling home-making and child-rearing at the same time. Others have active social lives with many late nights and they may be smoking and/or drinking too, putting additional stress on the nervous and physical systems of the body.

Stress leads to tension and anxiety, with an increase in nervous system activity and extra demands placed on the kidneys to filter adrenaline, a stimulating hormone produced by the body in stressful situations.

Even children can suffer from stress due to situations such as school exams, peer pressure or bullying, or emotional conflicts due to disharmony in the home. Shock, anxiety, fear or emotional trauma all take their toll on physical health and sow the seeds for infection.

A certain amount of stress is considered healthy as it keeps the body and mind alert. However, when a person is subjected to constant high levels of stress the body becomes fatigued and body systems start to break down, increasing the chance of infection.

## Summary

There are many contributory causes that can lead to an attack of cystitis. For each person the combination is different but all cystitis sufferers will recognize some of the causes outlined above as playing a role in their attacks.

Study each one carefully and then turn to the next chapter on self-help to find positive remedies for each of these causative factors that can actively help you prevent cystitis.

CHAPTER 4

# Self-help for cystitis

*How you can help yourself by minimizing or preventing the causes of cystitis*

Self-help is the key to preventing cystitis. All of the causative factors mentioned in the previous chapter can be minimized, if not entirely eliminated, by prompt and effective self-help action.

Each of the different causative factors will be addressed, one by one, with an explanation of how they can be avoided.

***1 Hygiene***

The key to good hygiene is appropriate washing and toilet wiping.

*For females*

- Always wipe from front to back after going to the toilet.
- Wash your perineal area regularly. Use soap at the anus but never over the vaginal area. Wash gently without rubbing and pat dry with a clean, soft flannel kept separately.
- Never douche or use talcum powders, deodorants or perfumed soaps on this area.
- If you are a chronic cystitis sufferer carry out Angela Kilmartin's bottle washing procedure *every time* you pass a stool It is vital that you follow the instructions *exactly* as she describes them (*see* box). She has

numerous stories of people who did not follow the procedure correctly and thereby did not get the desired result.

**Bottle washing**

Use the following cleansing routine after every bowel movement.

1 Wipe bottom from front to back with uncoloured, unscented toilet paper.
2 Stand up and wash hands under running, hot water at the basin.
3 Re-soap one hand with non-perfumed soap and soap anal area (not vaginal area) with it.
4 Rinse hand thoroughly.
5 Fill a 500 ml bottle, or two, with warm water. Return and sit on lavatory with backbone pointed down and pour water from the front slowly. Use the other hand to help clean off all the soap.
6 Pat dry with a soft flannel and keep it separate.

For full details of bottle washing procedures in different situations see Angela Kilmartin's book, *Cystitis; How to prevent infection and inflammation* (Thorsons, 1994).

*For children and babies*

- Change nappies regularly, at least every four hours, and always wipe female babies from front to back. Clean gently and thoroughly with clean cotton wool dipped in warm water.
- Teach young girls to wipe themselves from front to back and teach all children to wash their hands well after going to the toilet.
- Encourage children to go the toilet promptly when they feel the urge to urinate and to empty the bladder fully.

*For males*

- Always wash your hands after going to the toilet.
- Wash your penis regularly using mild soap and plain, warm water. Make sure to rinse under the foreskin as well. Cleanse gently.
- Wash the genitals and clean the hands and nails before sex. Keep fingernails short.

2 *Sex*

The majority of cystitis attacks that occur after sex could be completely prevented if only the following were always carried out.

- Always empty the bladder before sex.
- Wash the genital area gently with warm water before sex. Pat dry.
- Pass water as soon as possible after sex to eliminate any bacteria that may have entered the urethra. If necessary drink a glass of water before sex to ensure that you have some fluid to pass after love-making is finished.
- Make sure the vaginal passage is well lubricated to prevent bruising.
- Change position often to avoid excessive bruising in any one area.
- Cut nails short and keep them clean to prevent them harbouring and spreading germs.

Good hygiene before and after love-making, proper lubrication and gentle sex can all help prevent the spread of infection.

3 ***Vaginal health***

- Never douche. It destroys the delicate, natural balance of micro-organisms within the vagina.
- Use sanitary towels rather than tampons whenever possible, especially at night, as tampons have a very drying effect on the vagina. Change both regularly during the day, at least every four hours.

- Take care with your diet. Ensure it includes plenty of wholefoods and fresh vegetables. Avoid sugary and very spicy foods and too much citrus fruit. Drink plenty of water and avoid, or at least limit your intake of, coffee, tea and sugary, carbonated drinks.
- Promptly investigate and treat any vaginal infections.

Good vaginal health can be maintained by correct diet and good hygiene. Preventing infection in the vagina will also help to prevent infection spreading into the urethra.

*4 Digestion*

- Avoid constipation by ensuring you have plenty of fibre in your diet and drink plenty of water. Adding linseeds (available from health food shops) to your food can help too as they are rich in essential fatty acids which help to lubricate the large intestine.
- Ensure good digestion by eating a balanced diet, avoiding fast food and junk foods, chewing food well and taking time for meals.
- Check yourself for food allergies (*see* pages 66–7)
- If affected by *candida*, take probiotics and anti-fungals and follow the anti-candida diet (*see* pages 67–8)
- Cleansing fasts may also be beneficial (*see* page 83).

Good digestion, the prevention of constipation and elimination of foods to which your body is intolerant help prevent a build-up of bacteria in the gut that could spread out into the perineum.

*5 Position of bladder or uterus*

Regular exercise will ensure good muscle tone and firm support for the internal organs.

For females, pelvic floor exercises will keep the pelvic floor muscles strong, support the gynaecological organs and help control the flow of urine.

**Pelvic floor exercise**

- Cross your legs while standing or lying.
- Squeeze the pelvic muscles by pulling them up into the body, and hold. (Get a feel of these muscles by trying to stop and start the flow of urine when you go to the toilet but *always* make sure that you completely empty the bladder before finishing.
- Squeeze more and continue to hold.
- Squeeze even more and hold.
- Relax the muscles gradually, as if letting down a lift.
- Repeat often throughout the day for a minute or so at any time.

Oriental exercises such as yoga and *chi kung* can also be used to strengthen urinary function. Basically they work by stimulating the bladder and kidney meridians that course the back and the legs. One example is given below. For more details consult a yoga therapist or Robert Munroe's excellent book *Yoga for Common Ailments* (Gaia Books, London, 1994).

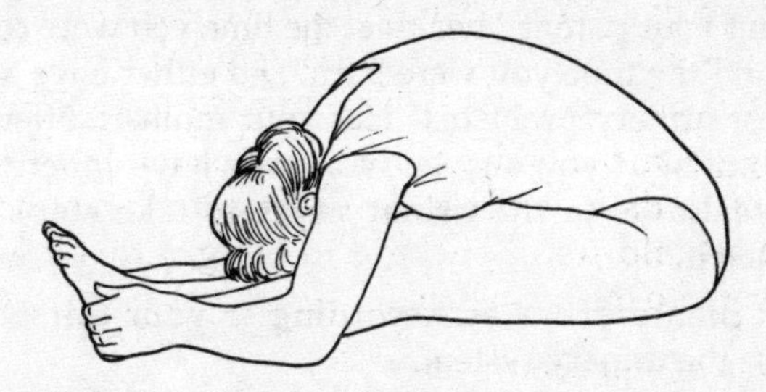

**Fig. 2 Forward bending pose (*Paschimottanasana*)**

Sit on the floor with the legs outstretched, relax the body and breathe deeply. Stretch the arms above the head as you inhale and then exhale while slowly bending forward from the waist. Keep the back straight and grasp the legs under the knees, by the ankles or at the toes, depending on your flexibility. Do not force or strain. Hold the stretch for a minute, breathing deeply, relaxing and increasing the stretch on each exhalation. Inhaling, slowly return to the starting position.

This exercise stimulates the bladder and kidney meridians in the back and legs and helps regulate urinary function.

**6 *Toilet training***

- Never try to retain urine. Go to the toilet at regular intervals and whenever you feel the need. This ensures that the urethra is flushed out at regular intervals and that no stale urine is retained in the bladder.
- Encourage children, especially young girls, to develop regular toilet habits and to not try to delay going to the toilet.
- Change babies' nappies promptly, and toddlers' underwear as soon as possible after any leakage, to prevent any infection or irritation developing.

**7 *Congenital weakness***

Check out your parents' health at the time you were conceived and the time you were born. Did either have any kidney or urinary problems? Has your mother suffered from cystitis? If you suspect you may have inherited some weakness in the urinary system take steps to strengthen it.

- Drink plenty of water, according to your thirst, to cleanse the urinary system.
- Eat plenty of pulses, especially aduki beans, and long white radish (known as 'mooli' or 'daikon'). According to macrobiotic principles these strengthen the kidneys and improve urinary function.
- Learn acupressure points that strengthen the kidneys and bladder (*see* pages 57–9). Meridian exercises and certain yoga postures may help too.

- Try acupuncture, shiatsu or reflexology to constitutionally strengthen the urogenital organs and improve urinary function. (*See* Chapters 7 and 10 on appropriate treatments and how to find a qualified practitioner.)

*8 Contraception*

- If you think you may be allergic or sensitive to the contraception you are using see your family doctor, or visit your local family planning clinic, to discuss alternatives. There is a wide range of contraceptives available and a change may make a big difference. For example, some creams used in combination with the cap may be less irritating than others.
- Alternatively, if you have a regular partner, consider natural fertility awareness as your chosen method of contraception, thereby avoiding all potential irritants. This method is based on a thorough understanding of precisely when ovulation occurs, using awareness of temperature and mucus changes during the menstrual cycle. If the method is learnt properly, practised for several months in conjunction with another method of contraception, and then carried out accurately it is an extremely effective form of birth control.

*9 Irritants*

Avoid all irritants that may enter the urethra.

- Use only mild soap for washing.
- Avoid strongly perfumed bath or shower products.
- Use non-biological soap powders.
- Rinse underwear by hand in plain water after washing them.
- Wear only 100 per cent cotton underwear or no underwear in warm weather.
- Avoid tight, restrictive clothing on the pelvis, such as tight jeans or nylons, to allow air to circulate in the perineal area.

- Always use a clean flannel when washing.
- Never use vaginal douches.

Avoid all irritants that may enter the blood stream via the mouth and the digestive system. The following are common irritants.

- Food additives and colourings
- Very spicy foods
- Very acidic foods and drinks such as sweets, coffee, tea, colas.

If necessary have yourself tested for allergens (*see* Chapter 7).

***10 Diet***

The general principle for a diet that prevents cystitis is to eat a balanced, wholefood diet with plenty of vegetables and to drink plenty of good quality water. Such a diet is basically alkaline in nature and this helps to maintain the neutral pH of the urine. Certain nutritional supplements may also be helpful if the diet is inadequate. Diet and nutrition are so important for cystitis that a complete chapter has been devoted to them (*see* Chapter 9).

***11 Posture***

There are many things you can try to improve your posture, and thereby improve your circulation and the drainage of blood and lymph in the pelvic region.

- Exercise regularly to improve muscle tone. Aerobic movement, gym work, stretching exercises and yoga are all beneficial. Swimming can be good too but be wary of highly chlorinated pools and make sure you change promptly once you are out of the water. Avoid getting chilled or remaining in a wet swimsuit for long.
- Stand tall and check the alignment of your pelvis whenever you are standing. Neither the stomach nor the buttocks should protrude excessively.

- If you work at a desk check your seating posture. If the angle of the seat of the chair cannot be adjusted then buy, or make, a wedge that will widen the angle that the thighs make with the hips. This prevents congestion of blood and lymph in the pelvic area. (Wedges are available from orthopaedic stockists or from many manipulative therapists.) Alternatively, specially designed orthopaedic chairs are a worthwhile investment for both your back and internal organs if you spend many hours every day at a desk.
- If your bed is more than ten years old consider replacing it or at least buying a new mattress. Poor support during the many hours spent sleeping can gradually weaken muscles and contribute to poor posture.
- For advice on exercises to improve posture consult a teacher of the Alexander Technique or an osteopath (*see* Chapter 7).

*12 Environment*

Avoid exposing the pelvic region to extremes of temperature and keep the lower regions of the body warm.

- Never sit on heaters or radiators or cold floors.
- Always change out of wet clothing as soon as possible, especially swimsuits.
- Keep the lower back and the midriff covered. Avoid short tops that end at the waist as this can lead to the navel and the bladder, or the lower back and the kidneys, getting chilled.
- Don't walk barefoot on cold floors. Wear slippers or mules.
- Keep the feet and ankles warm in winter.

*13 Medication*

If an attack of cystitis is already under way it may be necessary for you to take antibiotics to eradicate the infection. If so, always follow the procedure below.

- Ask your family doctor to test your urine to determine precisely which bacteria are present (*see* Chapter 5).
- Unless the attack is very severe, have your physician wait for the test results before prescribing the antibiotic. That way you can be sure you have the most effective and appropriate antibiotic for your infection.
- Always take the tablets with food and precisely as indicated. Always complete the course even if the symptoms subside, otherwise resistant bacteria may develop.
- After the course is complete take a course of *probiotics* to re-establish the balance of micro-organisms in the gut and help to prevent thrush. These should contain *Lactobacillus acidophilus* and *Bifidobacterium bifidus* and are available from most health food stores. The live, powdered product, which is kept refrigerated, is best. Take it as indicated for four weeks.

***14 Stress***

If you think stress and anxiety may play a role in your cystitis or may aggravate your symptoms then try the following.

- Re-evaluate your daily schedule. Are you doing too much? Could you prune your activities, share chores or delegate work?
- Make some time for rest and relaxation every day.
- Release all worries and tension before you go to sleep at night. Writing worries down on a piece of paper may help you to prioritize your affairs and develop solutions. Talking anxieties over with a friend or partner is also better than bottling things up.
- Exercise helps to release physical tension and relax the mind.
- If you feel you have psychological or sexual problems related to cystitis arrange to see a professionally trained therapist or counsellor (*see* Chapter 8).

- If young cystitis sufferers appear to be under emotional stress then help to create a loving, secure environment where they can express their feelings and get your help in working through problems.

### *15 Support groups*

Don't suffer alone. Many countries now have information and advice associations relating to cystitis and support groups for sufferers. Check out if there is something near you or even consider starting one yourself. Given the statistics there is bound to be someone suffering from cystitis in your street and many people in your neighbourhood. Why not help inform one another about all these self-help measures for prevention, support each other in educating family doctors and partners about cystitis, and help each other make the life changes that will eliminate the misery of cystitis from your life altogether?

### *16 Emergency self-help*

As soon as you feel the symptoms of cystitis you must take immediate action to stop any infection developing. Whatever you do, do not just lie down or go to sleep and hope the symptoms will go away. They will not. They will only get worse, so the sooner you take action the sooner you can get any infection under control and prevent it spreading.

The following First Aid procedure should be started immediately and continued until symptoms abate or until you can get to a doctor and have your urine tested. If you can, be prepared by making up a Cystitis First Aid Kit in advance and keep it handy in case of need. Otherwise do the best you can to follow the procedure described below with what you have available.

**Cystitis First Aid Kit**

1 **Urine specimen jar** (for urine sample – available from doctor's surgeries or pharmacies) or **heat-proof Pyrex jug and small, glass jar** with secure lid.
2 **Sodium bicarbonate powder** (available from pharmacies and the baking section in most supermarkets) or a box of sachets of an **alkalizing agent** (available over the counter – *see* page 40 for examples of brand names).
3 **Mild herbal teas** such as camomile (available loose from herbalists or in tea bags from health food stores and supermarkets) to calm the nerves and soothe irritation. **Parsley**, grown outside or on the windowsill is handy to have as a natural diuretic too.
4 A stock of **cranberry juice**, or **cranberry extract tablets**, and **lemon barley water** (unsweetened, low sugar or home made).
5 **Herbal remedies** such as bearberry or goldenseal in dried or tablet form (*see* page 74) and **homoeopathic remedies** such as Cantharsis 30c (*see* page 80). Also Echinacea (tablets or tincture), to help boost immunity.
6 **Bach Flower Rescue Remedy** drops (*see* page 97) which will help you cope with the pain and ease the trauma of cystitis.

The emergency self-help regimes in many books on cystitis focus solely on the bladder. The aim is to dilute the urine, increase the flow of urine and soothe irritation. Yet there are other things that it is also vital to do.

- Boost immune function in order to increase the body's resistance to infection.
- Make some dietary changes in order to reduce the acidity of the urine once the effect of the emergency alkalizing agents has worn off.
- Ensure good nutritional status to boost immunity and help the body fight infection.

- Address the causes of the cystitis in order to prevent re-infection.
- Strengthen yourself psychologically to cope with the cystitis.

The First Aid procedure described below will enable you to do all these. It is unique in that it combines the best of orthodox medicine, self-help procedures and natural remedies in order to help you overcome the cystitis and boost your health.

**First Aid for cystitis**

1 Prepare a **mid-stream urine sample** (*see* box on page 35) to be sent for testing. Take it early in the morning and do *not* drink beforehand as this will dilute the sample. Follow the instructions carefully to ensure the sample is not contaminated. **Refrigerate the sample immediately** and take to your doctor or laboratory for testing as soon as possible.

2 **Start drinking** to dilute your urine and make it less painful when you go to the toilet. Angela Kilmartin, author of several self-help guides for cystitis, recommends that you drink **half a pint (10fl.oz/250ml) of water straight away and another half a pint every 20 minutes for three hours**, and that this should be followed exactly for best results. She further recommends that in the initial half pint, and in the ones taken on the second and third hour, you **add** either **one level teaspoon of bicarbonate of soda or a sachet of an alkalizing agent from a pharmacy** (*see* page 40). (Follow the instructions on the packet.)
*Note*: Do not use bicarbonate of soda if you have any history of heart problems. Discontinue using it if you get palpitations or discomfort in the chest. As an alternative try Mist Pot Cit, a liquid potassium citrate mixture, available from any pharmacy, **or a herbal alternative** (*see* pages 74–5).

3 **Use natural diuretics** such as infusions of parsley, cranberry juice or watermelon to help flush the bladder. Many self-help regimes recommend taking a cup of strong coffee on the hour every hour for the first three hours. This will certainly have a diuretic effect but it will also irritate the bladder further. Herbal diuretics are less irritating and therefore preferable if you have them available (*see* pages 74–5).
4 **Make yourself as comfortable as you can.** Keep warm and rest. If you have hot water bottles you can place them on your abdomen and your back and tuck yourself up in bed or in an armchair. Alternatively, you may find a **sitz bath** (hip-bath) helpful (*see* page 84).
5 **To relieve the pain** and help you cope use a herbal sedative such as **camomile tea** (*see* page 32), **homoeopathic remedies** (*see* page 78 ff.), or an **aromatherapy oil** rubbed into the abdomen or added to the bath (*see* page 61). Placing a few drops of the **Bach Flower Rescue Remedy** (*see* page 96) in a glass of water and sipping it throughout the day will also help you to deal with the shock and trauma of having cystitis. If you really feel you need them you can use painkillers but these are not ideal as they will mask the body's signals and can also suppress immune function. It is better if you can be fully aware of what is going on in your body and take an active part in your recovery.
6 Utilize some of the **natural self-help remedies** such as **acupressure** (*see* pages 57–9) to strengthen bladder and kidney function, **aromatherapy oils** (*see* page 63) as natural antiseptics and for calming, **herbal remedies** (*see* page 72 ff.) to reduce inflammation and aid urination, **homoeopathic remedies** (*see* page 80) to reduce symptoms and trigger the body's healing mechanisms and **Flower Remedies** (*see* pages 96, 97) to improve your state of mind.
7 **Improve your diet.** Cut out all sweets, refined carbohydrates, meat, alcohol, tea and coffee. Follow the recommendations for a **healthy diet** on page 101 and

start the **anti-candida diet** (page 68) straight away if you also have thrush and feel *candida* may be a problem too. This will help speed up your recovery and decrease the likelihood of re-infection. **Fasting** may also be helpful (*see* page 83) but get expert advice on this.

8 **Improve your nutritional status.** 500 mg of Vitamin C (buffered types are less acidic) taken every two hours will help your body fight infection. Supplements of Vitamins A and E, B complex, essential fatty acids and zinc and a course of probiotics may also be helpful, especially if you are run-down. *See* the guidelines on page 102 and get specialist advice if you are pregnant.

9 **Stay positive.** You will get through the cystitis and you will learn a lot about your body and how to stay healthy in the process. Use mental affirmations to keep your spirits up (*see* page 90).

**How to take a mid-stream urine sample (MSU)**

1 Prepare a sterilized container to collect the urine and a smaller sterilized container to store it. To do this pour boiling water from the kettle into any heat-proof jug, or large jar, and into a smaller glass jar or specimen jar placed in the sink. Shake them dry rather than wiping them with a cloth which may contaminate them. Cover the containers with a clean cloth and take them to the bathroom.
*Note*: Sterilized urine specimen jars can be obtained from any doctor's surgery or pharmacy. If you have been prone to cystitis keep one handy at home in case of need.

2 While squatting, gently clean your perineal area with moist cotton wool balls or a clean flannel. Do not dry. (Males should clean the penis with water and a clean flannel and then proceed from point 4).

3 Clean the toilet seat with water and a mild cream cleanser (not disinfectant) and sit far back on it to allow space for the jug, or jar, when you take the sample.

4 Pass a small amount of urine into the toilet and then stop mid-stream.
5 Place your sterile container at the opening of the urethra and pass some urine into it.
6 Remove the container and empty the remainder of your bladder in the toilet.
7 Transfer the urine into the smaller container and seal it. Clean up and label the container with your name, your doctor's name and the date and time of the sample.
8 Refrigerate the sample until it can be delivered for analysis. Get it to your doctor or laboratory as soon as possible.

By following this approach you will feel much better within two to three hours. The pain will decrease, the spread of bacteria will be halted and your health and wellbeing will improve. You will be in a better position to prevent re-infection and you may avoid the need for antibiotics. (However, always get the results of your urine test, and have a follow-up test if necessary, to ensure that all bacteria have been eradicated, otherwise re-infection will occur.) This approach is simple and inexpensive, and it works!

*Note:* For further self-help tips see the natural therapies chapters.

CHAPTER 5

# Conventional treatments and procedures

If you suspect you have cystitis you should:

- start emergency self-help measures immediately (*see* pages 31–6)
- prepare a mid-stream urine sample for testing (*see* pages 35–6)
- consult your family doctor as soon as possible, arranging to have your urine sample tested and to collect a prescription as necessary

## Urine samples and urine testing

In healthy adults and children the urine is sterile so a mid-stream urine (MSU) sample can be used to test for the presence of bacteria. It is crucial to take the urine sample correctly to avoid contamination or an unrepresentative sample.

The sample is then sent to a laboratory for microscopy (examination under a microscope), culture (the bacteria are given optimal conditions to develop overnight and then rechecked) and sensitivity (where the bacteria's response to various antibiotics is checked). The whole process takes 48–72 hours.

In microscopy the sample is checked visually for pus and blood cells, indicating inflammation; skin cells, indicating contamination of the sample; or crystals, indicating kidney problems. Following overnight culture the sample is checked for the different types and numbers of bacteria.

The groups of bacteria responsible for cystitis are principally the *Coliform* group, consisting of *Escherichia (E. coli), Klebsiella* and *Proteus* and the *Coccus* group consisting of *Pseudomonas, Staphylococcus* and *Streptococcus.* The majority of positive samples show the presence of *E. coli* and *Streptococcus faecalis* bacteria. All of these bacteria are present in our large intestine and faeces.

The presence of more than 100,000 organisms per millilitre in the urine sample is considered evidence of a urinary tract infection. Your test result will name the offending bacteria and also indicate whether the growth is heavy, medium or insignificant.

An MSU is usually sufficient to confirm an infection but if there is uncertainty a urine culture may be obtained by bladder catheterization for further examination.

### Differentiating cystitis from other urogenitary conditions

If the doctor wants to distinguish between a vaginal, urethral or bladder infection for a female patient then a swab from the vaginal opening and a urethral urine sample (the first urine that is expelled) may be taken as well. In men, samples of prostate fluid and urethral urine may also be taken to distinguish between urethral, bladder and prostate infections. To obtain the prostate sample the gland is massaged and then the fluid expressed through the penis. Comparison of the samples is used to determine the seat of infection.

### Sensitivity plates

When samples are found to be positive for bacterial infection, sensitivity plates are set up to establish which antibiotic will best treat the infection. Small numbers of organisms are taken from the sample and left overnight on plates impregnated with different antibiotics known to be effective against urinary infections. The antibiotics are divided into groups known to be effective against different types of bacteria.

By the next morning the organisms will have grown around some of the antibiotics but not others. It is these others which will then be used in treatment.

### Commonly prescribed medication

If the cystitis is found to be non-bacterial, and kidney function is normal, you will normally be prescribed drugs that are alkalizing agents. These are also available over the counter in most countries. These drugs are potassium or sodium based and work by raising the pH of the urine, making it more alkaline. This stops the burning sensation of acidic urine and provides symptomatic relief. Alternatively pharmacists can be asked to make up Mist Pot Cit, a liquid potassium citrate mixture that is far cheaper than the branded alkalizing agents but just as effective.

If the cystitis is bacterial then antibacterial or antibiotic drugs are required. The antibacterials, known as quinolones, act by inhibiting the enzyme that maintains the DNA structure of the bacteria and this prevents them multiplying. Antibiotics are antibacterial substances derived from fungi and bacteria and are classified according to the spectrum of bacteria they can eradicate.

## Medication for cystitis

**Alkalizing agents (available over the counter)**

| | |
|---|---|
| *Cystemme** | Sodium bicarbonate plus sodium citrate |
| *Cystopurin** | Potassium citrate plus sweetener |
| *Cystitis Relief** | Sodium citrate plus sweetener and flavouring |
| *Effercitrate** | Potassium citrate |

**Quinolones**

| | |
|---|---|
| *Nalidixic acid*, *Norfloxacin* | Used for both acute and chronic urinary infection |
| *Nitrofurantoin* | An antibacterial used for urinary infections where the urine is highly acidic. Interferes with bacterial DNA. Can be used during early stages of pregnancy. |
| *Fosfomycin* | Often used as a single dose treatment for acute and uncomplicated infections of the lower urinary tract. It is antibacterial, with a broad spectrum of activity, and acts by breaking down the bacterial cell walls. |
| *Hexamine* | An antibacterial sometimes used in long-term treatment for recurrent infections, especially with the elderly. Only effective with acid urine and often causes side-effects |

**Antibiotics**

| | |
|---|---|
| *Amoxil** | A broad spectrum penicillin |
| *Macrobid** | A sustained release nitrofurantoin used for urinary tract infections |
| *Macrodantin** | A nitrofurantoin used for urinary tract infections |
| *Mictral**, *Negram** | Quinolones containing nalidixic acid used for acute urinary infections |
| *Trimopan** | A trimethoprim product commonly used for acute urinary infections |
| *Utinor** | A quinolone containing norfloxacin and used for acute, chronic and complicated urinary infections |

*Note:* Asterisks refer to brand names used in the UK

Drugs are known by both their generic names and their brand names. Their generic name is the same the world over but brand names vary from country to country. One of the most commonly prescribed drugs for cystitis is trimethoprim which is sold under many different brand names and available in tablet form for adults and in liquid form for children. (Typical dosage is 200mg twice a day for adults and half that for children aged six to twelve.) Amoxycillin (marketed as Amoxil in the UK and as Larotid and Polymox in the USA) is also widely used for infections of the lower urinary tract. (Typical dosage is 250–500 mg three times a day for adults and half dosage for children aged three to ten years.) Dosages vary according to age and body size and are always substantially reduced for children and infants.

If a vaginal swab was taken and showed the presence of *candida* or *chlamydia*, or if you have a history of developing thrush when you take antibiotics, you may also be prescribed oral and/or vaginal anti-fungal medication such as Nystatin (UK brand name, known as Mycostatin in the USA and Australia).

You may be prescribed medication for three, five, seven or ten days duration. Discuss this with your doctor and then take as directed and complete the course. If you do not, any remaining bacteria may start to multiply again causing re-infection or they may develop resistance to the antibiotic.

## Drug safety

When high levels of bacteria are found in a urine sample it is essential to treat the infection with antibacterial or antibiotic drugs in order to prevent the infection spreading up to the kidneys, which can cause permanent damage or can even be fatal. However, drugs also often cause side-effects so you should be sure to inform yourself as much as possible about the drug and take it exactly as prescribed and for the recommended duration.

Just because a drug is prescribed it does not mean it is safe. It can be many years before all the possible side-effects are known. One example is the drug co-trimoxazole (sulphamethoxazole plus trimethoprim), marketed as Septrin in the UK, Septra in the USA and Trib in Australia. This drug was used widely for urinary infections for many years, especially with the elderly, even though there was never one single study carried out on its long-term effects in elderly patients. More recently it has declined in popularity after being linked with liver and kidney damage.

### Other medical investigations

Your doctor may want to do further tests to check the functioning of the kidneys and bladder. These may include the following.

- **Catheterization** – A fine tube (catheter) is inserted to take urine samples directly from the ureters and kidneys.
- **Cystometry (urodynamic studies)** – a series of measurements taken while filling and emptying the bladder to evaluate bladder function.
- **Endoscopy** – a fibre-optic tube is inserted, under sedation or anaesthetic, to allow the lining of the urethra (**urethroscopy**) and the bladder (**cystoscopy**) to be viewed.
- **Intra-venous pyelogram (IVP)** – X-ray of the kidneys and ureter after dye has been injected.
- **Micturating cystogram** – an X-ray of the bladder taken during urination.

These tests are used to rule out problems such as kidney stones, stenosis (narrowing of the ureters), reflux (backward flow of urine due to faulty valves), cysts, polyps and tumours. If tumours of the kidney or prostate are suspected you may also be given an **ultrasound scan**, a **computerized axial tomography (CAT) scan** or be sent for **nuclear magnetic resonance (NMR)** imaging (known as **MRI** in the USA).

### Surgical treatment

Apart from drugs you may also be offered surgical treatment. This can include the following.

- **Dilatation** – Stretching or enlarging the urethra or bladder.
- **Cauterization** – Heat treatment to burn away infected or scarred tissue in the urethra or bladder.

There is no guarantee that these treatments will prevent cystitis; and surgery, involving anaesthetic and post-operative recovery, should never be considered lightly. Always fully inform yourself about the procedure involved and discuss the risks and likely benefits with your consultant.

### Other treatments

Some doctors have been developing their own treatments for cystitis using intravenous hydrogen peroxide to reduce inflammation or intravesical BCG (Bacillus Calmette-Guérin, an attenuated strain of bovine tuberculosis bacterium) to enhance immune function. However, the numbers of people receiving such treatments are very small and there have been no long-term studies of their effects, so caution should be exercised.

CHAPTER 6

# Natural therapies and cystitis

*Introducing the gentle alternatives*

Although cystitis is most commonly treated with a combination of self-help measures and medical intervention, if the infection is acute, many sufferers have found natural therapies to be very beneficial too. These therapies can help you break out of the cycle of recurrent cystitis, antibiotics and thrush and help to improve your general health and wellbeing at the same time.

The so-called 'natural therapies' are mostly based on long-standing traditions of healing and medicine from both East and West. In essence they are not new, although they may include modern developments, but have been tried and tested over the centuries. It is worth remembering that modern medicine, as we know it, has only been around for a few hundred years and that many of the Western medical drugs used today are actually based on plant and herbal extracts.

The popularity of natural therapies is increasing all the time. A recent *Which?* report found that one in eight people in the UK have consulted a practitioner of natural therapies at some time and a large proportion reported high levels of satisfaction and significant improvements in their conditions. A British Medical Association report in 1993 also conceded that the therapies could be beneficial and should become more widely available.

## Narrowing the gap with orthodox medicine

Many medical doctors are now informing themselves about natural therapies and even training in them. The standards of training for the natural therapies have also improved dramatically in recent years and extensive cover of Western medicine is often included. A gradual increase in good quality research into natural therapies is also helping to establish their efficacy.

Already there are many examples of practitioners of Western medicine and of natural therapies working alongside one another in hospitals and clinics for the benefit of patients. As a result the gap between the two is narrowing and it is no longer appropriate to suggest that the two are in conflict with one another. Rather, it would seem that an integrated approach with the best of modern medicine and appropriate natural therapies combined with health education and self-help measures may be the best way forward.

## Why use natural therapies?

Many people are turning to natural therapies because they want to take more responsibility for their own health, because of a preference for a non-drug and more holistic approach or because they are disenchanted with modern medical practices. They may be unhappy with short consultation times, long waiting lists for treatment and a heavy reliance on drugs. Or they may be concerned about the possible side-effects of drugs following heavy publicity about certain drugs that have gone catastrophically wrong, such as thalidomide. There are also certain basic principles underlying natural therapy which many people find attractive.

## The principles of natural therapies

The core principle of natural therapies is that the person as a whole, and as an individual, is treated rather than the symptom or disease. A practitioner of natural therapy would therefore focus not only on your cystitis but also on your general heath and vitality, diet, lifestyle, etc and each person's treatment is individual.

The following are generally held to be common features of natural therapies.

- A symptom or disease is regarded as a sign that the body is out of balance. Treatment aims to restore the overall balance of the vital organs and body metabolism.
- True health is regarded as a balanced body, mind and spirit and not just the removal of symptoms. Treatment is not only aimed at the physical level but at the emotional, mental and spiritual levels too.
- The body is believed to have its own innate ability to heal itself. Therapy aims to stimulate this natural ability.
- The secret of success lies in determining and treating the underlying cause of the condition. The presenting symptom may be just the most recent, and surface, sign of imbalance. It is important to treat the root cause that brought it about in the first place.
- Every person is individual and should be treated as such. No person's treatment will be exactly the same as anyone else's.
- The individual plays an important role in healing. The therapist is the instrument rather than the doer. As the individual takes more personal responsibility for his or her own health, so healing becomes more effective and more permanent.
- Social and environmental factors also play an important role in health and disease. The person's life situation should be considered along with the symptoms.

- The mental aspect is important. If a person can understand his or her imbalance and think positively about his or her health, this will facilitate healing.
- Treatments used should be as gentle as possible, activating the body's natural healing ability, and not causing harm.
- Therapists should be self-aware and take responsibility for their own health in order to be able to facilitate healing in others.
- There is a universal, cosmic energy, the power of creation and of nature, divine power manifest in material phenomena, which can be drawn on to empower healing. Good practitioners from any discipline utilize this consciously or unconsciously.

**How natural therapies treat cystitis**

Natural therapies are ideal for treating someone suffering from cystitis as they can help to:

- relieve or remove symptoms of urinary discomfort
- strengthen the urinary system
- promote healing of scar tissue
- boost immunity and increase the ability to fight infection
- address the psychological and emotional components of cystitis by helping to reduce anxiety and fear
- promote general health, vitality and wellbeing

The approaches of different therapies vary. Some will focus more on the physical body. Osteopathy, for example, may help promote circulation and drainage of blood and lymph in the pelvic region thereby assisting good function of the bladder and kidneys. Other therapies work more energetically. For example, an acupuncturist treating someone with cystitis may insert needles in the ankles, legs and back in order to improve the flow of vital energy within the acupuncture meridians – lines of electrical energy – corresponding to the kidney and bladder. Other therapies may aim to treat the body via the power of the mind. For example, hypnotherapy may help to address fears and anxieties related to cystitis and can help you to develop a positive mental image about your health.

## Do natural therapies work?

The amount of scientific research into natural therapies is increasing every year. Many of the studies have had encouraging results and back up the anecdotal reports over hundreds, if not thousands, of years of the potential benefits of such treatments.

The number of studies focusing on cystitis is limited but Chinese studies have shown clear effects of acupuncture on the urinary system and herbal studies have demonstrated the efficacy of plants such as cranberry in improving urinary function. These are discussed in more detail in the next chapter.

More funding, research training and investigation of new research methods are required but it is surely only a matter of time before the therapies are better understood and more widely employed in current medical care.

## Choosing a therapy

There are so many therapies on offer, it is easy to become overwhelmed and not know where to start. Some therapies, such as acupuncture, are complete systems of medicine in their own right, while others involve a specific set of techniques for addressing imbalance. Many therapies now have well established training institutions and procedures and professional associations with rigorous codes of conduct and ethics. These have helped to raise the profile of the therapies and have increased public confidence in both the service providers and the services being offered.

In many countries it is becoming possible to receive natural therapy under the national health systems or under the cover of private medical insurance. For example, in some European countries homeopathy is part of the state system; in the UK increasing numbers of Health Service Trusts and fund-holding medical practices are buying in the services of natural therapists; and in some states in the USA insurance companies are required to cover the cost of treatments such as acupuncture.

Some of the therapies have proven effectiveness while others have only anecdotal reports of benefits, although the numbers of reports may be very large. The following are important points to remember when choosing a therapy.

- Find out as much as you can about the therapy concerned to see if you think it will suit you.
- Always ensure that the practitioner you see is properly qualified. (*See* Chapter 10 on how to find and choose a natural therapist.) Personal recommendation is also helpful.
- Check if the practitioner has experience of treating cystitis, what the treatment will involve, what results would be expected and how many treatment sessions are likely to be needed.
- Check out the financial implications. Is the therapy covered by insurance or available within the State system? If you find you have to pay for the therapy yourself the cost may appear daunting, but consider the fact that it will be a worthwhile investment if it really helps you to transform your health for the better.

- Don't expect the therapy to provide a miracle cure but do expect positive results. If there is no improvement after a full course of treatment it may be that this particular therapy is not helpful for you and you need to consider something else. However do be aware that:

  Natural therapies sometimes work slowly. Give your body time to respond, and complete the course of treatment rather than giving up in the early stages.

  Symptoms can sometimes get worse before they get better. This is known as the 'healing crisis' as the body activates healing mechanisms to fight disease and infection. This phenomenon is accepted with therapies such as homeopathy, acupuncture or herbal medicine and is nothing to be alarmed about. However, do keep in contact with your therapist as it may be necessary to adjust your treatment according to your body's response.

- Monitor your condition and take an active role in your treatment, following carefully any guidance given.
- Keep your family doctor informed of any treatment you are undergoing.

### Which therapies may be helpful?

For the purposes of clarity the therapies covered in this book have been divided into those that work principally via the body and those that work mainly through the mind and emotions. It should be remembered, however, that this is really just a convenience as there is considerable overlap between the two. Acupuncture, for example, may directly improve bladder and kidney function but as you start to feel more vitality and wellbeing you will feel happier and more confident and relaxed too and this, in turn, will lead to improved circulation and greater physical wellbeing.

The therapies covered by this book are listed below and the next three chapters describe the role they can play in helping you to stop cystitis and permanently prevent its recurrence.

**Natural therapies for cystitis**

**Treating the body (Chapter 7)**
Acupuncture
Acupressure
Alexander Technique
Aromatherapy
Clinical ecology (allergy testing)
Healing
Herbal medicine
Homeopathy
Massage
Naturopathy
Osteopathy and Chiropractic
Reflexology

**Treating the mind (Chapter 8)**
Cognitive therapy
Counselling and Psychotherapy
Flower remedies
Hypnotherapy
Meditation
Relaxation training
Sexual therapy

**Diet and nutrition (Chapter 9)**
Dietary therapy
Nutritional therapy

All of these therapies are practised by qualified professionals but many also incorporate First Aid and self-help treatments that can be used by anyone. These are included in the following chapters. If you decide to use these please remember to make the following checks.

- Fully familiarize yourself with the procedure or remedy before carrying it out or taking it.
- Follow the directions given exactly.
- Obtain the name of a qualified practitioner in the appropriate speciality whom you can contact if you have any doubts or problems. (*See* Appendix A: Useful Organizations.)

CHAPTER 7

# Treating the body

*Physical therapies for cystitis*

This chapter describes the natural therapies that can help you to heal yourself by strengthening the physical body and improving the functioning of the vital organs. Although the focus may be on a physical level there really is no separation of mind and body so there are bound to be psychological effects also.

With cystitis, these therapies focus on improving the functioning of the bladder and kidneys, improving circulation of blood and lymph, increasing the health of the tissues and enhancing general health and vitality.

## Acupuncture

Acupuncture is one of the oldest and most widely used of the natural therapies. It is part of a complete medical system, that of Oriental medicine, and originated in China, Korea, Japan and Tibet. It is widely practised in the Far East to this day and is increasingly popular in Europe, North America and Australasia. It is estimated that several million acupuncture consultations take place every working day, and the World Health Organization (WHO) has officially recognized more than one hundred medical complaints that can be improved or cured by acupuncture.

Acupuncture involves the insertion of fine needles into points on the body known as 'acupoints' which are said to lie along energetic pathways of the body known as 'meridians'. Although the meridians cannot be seen by the naked eye they have been demonstrated electrically, and thermographically using heat sensitive liquid crystals on the surface of the skin. Some healers claim to be able to 'feel' these pathways while sensitives have also reported being able to see them extrasensorily. They may also be felt subjectively, for example during an acupuncture treatment.

Some researchers have argued that the energy flowing through the meridians is electrical in nature. This fits well with descriptions in ancient Oriental medical texts of vital energy that flows through the meridians, powers the internal organs and is essential to life. According to Oriental medical theory, when there is plenty of vital energy flowing freely through the meridians there is good health. When the flow is blocked or impaired imbalance results and the corresponding internal organs will eventually become diseased.

A central tenet of Oriental medicine is the concept of prevention. If an imbalanced meridian can be treated in time, symptoms at an organic level may be prevented. In an acupuncture consultation the practitioner will diagnose your state of health using pulse diagnosis, observation of the tongue, palpation of different points on the body and questioning. On the basis of this diagnosis points will be selected for treatment to rebalance the flow of energy in the meridians and thereby improve health. Consultations generally last from 20 minutes to one hour.

If done correctly acupuncture is virtually painless, and during and after treatment comfortable sensations of relaxation and wellbeing are experienced which are thought to be due to the release of endorphins, the body's natural painkillers, into the bloodstream. All qualified acupuncturists use strict standards of hygiene and the majority now use disposable needles so there should be no risk of infection from the procedure.

Many acupuncturists also use adjunct therapies such as moxibustion (heat therapy), herbal medicine, massage, plum-blossom needling (a stimulatory technique) and cupping (a vacuum technique designed to increase circulation) as part of the treatment.

Studies investigating the effect of acupuncture on cystitis are currently underway in the West but several studies in China have already demonstrated improvement in urinary function after a course of acupuncture treatment. (A course generally consists of about ten treatments.)

The traditional Oriental medical view of cystitis is in terms of an accumulation of damp heat in the bladder. Treatment aims to dispel the damp and clear the heat. Points along the bladder meridian, on the ankles and back of the legs are often used together with abdominal points and points on the back (*see* Acupressure section below).

Acupuncture has been shown to help in the recovery of scar tissue externally so it may also promote healing of scar tissue internally.

**Summary:** Acupuncture can improve urinary function and reduce pain. It also helps to build general health and vitality.

**Carol's experience with acupuncture**

Carol, a 28-year-old bank clerk, had suffered from cystitis since she was a teenager. Since getting married two years earlier her attacks had been more frequent and more severe. She knew little about self-help techniques and had taken antibiotics every time she had cystitis.

As a child Carol had suffered from frequent sore throats and ear infections. She had had her tonsils removed when she was 14 but still occasionally got sore throats. Otherwise her health was good except that she complained of often feeling tired and having low back pain. The repeated cystitis was beginning to make her depressed and anxious and she was worried about the effect on her husband.

A friend recommended an acupuncturist to Carol and she decided to give it a try. Although she did not have cystitis at the time she went for acupuncture, the acupuncturist diagnosed weak kidneys and bladder function from Carol's pulses and tongue. The acupuncturist also explained to her that in Oriental medicine weak kidneys corresponded to ear and throat problems, back pain and tiredness as well as urinary problems. She told Carol that all of these should improve as her kidney vitality improved.

Carol went to see the acupuncturist every week for ten weeks. Fine needles were inserted in her ankles, wrists, abdomen and back and she was surprised how painless they were. She had been quite nervous, but after the first treatment she relaxed and began to look forward to the treatments. The acupuncturist also used heat treatment on her abdomen by lighting tiny cones of moxa wool and stopping them burning just before they reached the skin. Afterwards Carol's whole abdomen would feel warm and she would feel much more energetic.

As the treatments went on Carol's energy and vitality returned and she became much more cheerful once again. Her back pain and sore throats disappeared and she had no further bouts of cystitis. The acupuncturist also gave her some self-help books to read and she made some changes to her diet and hygiene. Six months later she was still free of cystitis and confident that it would not return.

Carol has continued to visit the acupuncturist twice a year for 'top-up' treatments 'because I always feel fantastic afterwards. The acupuncture has given me a new lease of life. I'm no longer plagued with cystitis or sore throats and I feel I have much more energy than before. Even my general health has improved and I never seem to catch whatever bug is going round at work. I'd recommend it to anyone and just wish I'd discovered it soon enough to prevent the years of misery I had with cystitis.'

**Acupressure**

Acupressure is really acupuncture without needles. Acupoints along meridian lines are selected for their effects on the urinary system but pressure is applied with a fingertip, or with the thumb, rather than a needle being inserted.

The beauty of acupressure is that anyone can practise it as it is safe and without side-effects. However, you must learn the point locations correctly for it to be effective and also familiarize yourself with contraindications. For example, certain points are not used during pregnancy as they promote labour. It is also important to know in which direction to apply pressure as this affects the flow of energy in the meridian.

There have been no scientific studies to date on the effect of acupressure on cystitis but many people report that it helps them prevent attacks. It is probably more useful for prevention than for cure and would not be sufficient treatment in the case of acute infection.

There is evidence that acupressure has been practised since ancient times in the Far East and also in Egypt. In countries such as Japan it is still widely used today, especially for the relief of tension and pain. If you want to do it yourself you can learn the points and techniques from an acupressure book but it may be easier to do a course to be sure you can locate the points correctly. If you would prefer someone to do it for you, try a shiatsu practitioner (*see* Shiatsu page 82 in this chapter and also Chapter 10) or, failing that, an acupuncturist. Most acupuncturists prefer to use needles but shiatsu practitioners work with their hands and fingers.

**Summary:** Acupressure may help in preventing cystitis. It is thought to strengthen bladder and kidney function.

### Alexander Technique

The Alexander Technique was devised in the 1920s by an actor, F Matthias Alexander, who developed problems with his breathing and speech. He began to notice that poor posture and muscle tension over many years caused physical function to deteriorate and he devised a set of exercises to 're-educate' the body to move correctly.

Alexander firmly believed that the body has a natural way of moving and that this can restore itself if old habits are corrected. He was particularly interested in the alignment of the head with the spine, and here his work has some overlap with the concepts of cranial

Apply perpendicular pressure to each point with the tip of the middle or index finger, or the thumb. Use small rotating movements for about 60 seconds, two or three times a day.

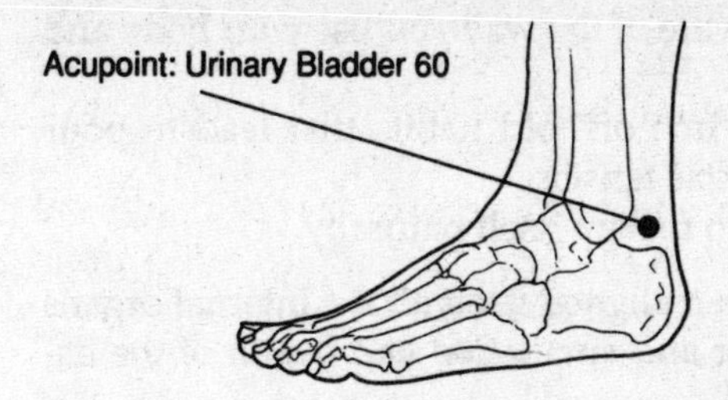


*Acupoint UB 60* On the outside of the ankle, half-way between the outside of the ankle bone and the Achilles tendon. Reduces pain and regulates bladder function.
*Caution*: Not to be used during pregnancy.

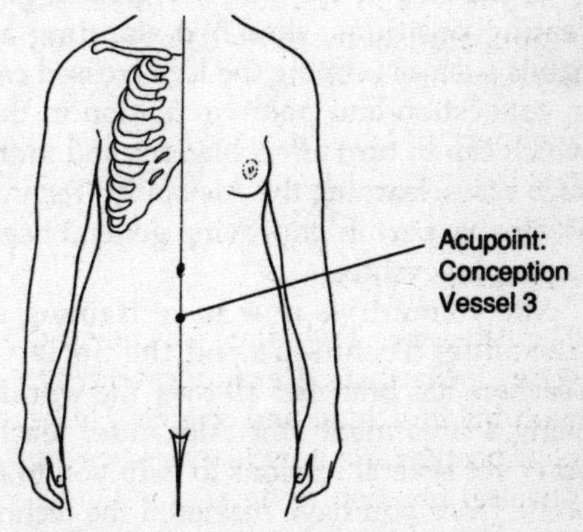


*Acupoint CV 3* On the abdominal mid line 4 thumb widths below the navel. Regulates bladder function and improves circulation around the abdominal organs. Helps to clear heat in the bladder.

**Fig. 3 Acupressure points for cystitis**

osteopathy (*see* Osteopathy section, pages 85–8), especially when moving from sitting to standing or lying down. The Alexander exercises therefore help you to:

- become more aware of the way you use your body and how you move
- help you to 'switch off' old habits that lead to poor posture and muscle tension
- allow the body to realign itself naturally

Once the body has realigned itself all the internal organs can function better and circulation and health of the tissues are improved.

The Alexander Technique concerns itself more with the whole body and its use than with specific physical symptoms but it is thought to be helpful for a wide range of physical problems that are posture-related.

In the case of cystitis poor general posture, hunched seating positions, slouched standing and bad sitting habits such as keeping the legs crossed can all contribute to congestion and poor circulation in the pelvic region which can in turn affect bladder and kidney function. In such cases, learning the Alexander Technique could play a valuable part in improving general health and helping to prevent cystitis.

Many countries now have training schools for the Alexander Technique and the Society of Alexander Teachers has branches all over the world. Rather than it being a 'treatment', the Alexander teacher works with you over several sessions to help you to re-educate your body. Once you have mastered the techniques you then keep practising them yourself in daily life.

There are no scientific studies of the effect of the Alexander Technique on cystitis but detailed studies by Dr W Barlow, a London physician, on musicians and actors using the technique all show marked improvement in posture and respiration and with minor problems such as back pain. People who have learnt the technique always look better and feel better and many report improvement in physical symptoms too. There are also sound physiological explanations for its effects in terms of the reactivation of dormant muscle spindles, the retraining of muscle groups so they are used more effectively and the co-ordinated signalling of reflexes to the brain. In this way the Alexander Technique can be understood as a technique that helps to harmonize both mind and body through optimizing posture and movement patterns.

**Summary:** The Alexander Technique improves posture and movement as well as mental and physical balance. It improves circulation and vitality in the pelvic region which may help urinary function.

### Aromatherapy

Aromatherapy uses the essential oils of plants which are applied to the body through massage, inhalation, compresses or baths. The actual term, 'aromatherapy' was first used in the 1920s by a Frenchman, Gattefossé, who studied the oils after accidentally discovering the healing power of lavender oil on a burn. The practice has been around since ancient times and was favoured by the Greeks and the Egyptians. Nowadays it is widely practised in France and is gaining in popularity in the UK.

The oils are carefully extracted from plants and then preserved. Once an essential oil has been absorbed into the body it is dispersed via the extra-cellular fluids. No one is certain exactly how the oils work but there is evidence that different oils stimulate activity in different centres of the brain, and the renowned aromatherapist, Robert Tisserand, has suggested that some are taken up by specific organs of the body.

Although aromatherapy is often thought of as a beauty treatment it is also considered to be helpful for a wide range of health problems. Oils commonly used for cystitis are listed in the box below. They can be applied either on a compress or by means of a few drops added to the bath water.

**Aromatherapy oils for cystitis**

**Bergamot** (not to be used if pregnant)

**Cedarwood** (Atlas, Texan and Virginian) (not to be used if pregnant)

**Camomile** (German and Roman)

**Lavender** (Spike and True)

**Sandalwood**

**Tea tree**

A qualified aromatherapist will help you select the most appropriate oil and advise you on the best way to use it. If you decide to use the oils by yourself *always* remember to consult the appropriate safety data. Oils are very powerful and some can irritate while others should never be taken internally. Some are contraindicated for pregnant women or babies.

When buying oils always buy the best. Don't be deceived by cheap, poor quality oils. The price depends on the method of preparation and this also influences its effectiveness. Research by prominent French aromatherapist Valnet has shown that chemically synthesized versions of the oils have very different properties to those of the real thing.

Also, never apply the oils directly on the skin unless with specialist advice. They should always be diluted in a carrier oil, such as almond oil, or added to water, for example in the bath.

Although there is a growing body of research into the properties of the oils themselves, and individual responses to them, there is little research into their effectiveness for specific ailments such as cystitis. Some of the oils' properties are particularly relevant for cystitis; for example, bergamot and cedarwood are antiseptic and diuretic while lavender is antiseptic and calming (although recent research by Baerheim and Scheffer has suggested that the diuretic effects of most oils are negligible).

Aromatherapy is probably most useful in the case of stress-related cystitis as it can help to relax and calm. It can thus be helpful in preventing cystitis and in getting you through the anxiety and stress of an acute infection. Essential oils are also excellent natural antiseptics.

A few drops of lavender oil in bath water will give you an aromatic and relaxing bath that is also naturally antiseptic. This will help keep the genital area free from bacteria thereby preventing infection (but remember never to soak in hot baths for long if you are a cystitis sufferer).

Oils applied on compresses and in sitz baths may also be helpful. (*See* box below and section on naturopathy, page 82.) In Europe they are also sometimes used for douches but cystitis sufferers are generally advised not to douche as this can dry natural secretions and make the problem worse.

**Summary:** Aromatherapy is good for stress-related cystitis; it helps to relax and calm. It is also excellent as a natural antiseptic, but may be insufficient in the case of acute infection.

### Using aromatherapy for cystitis

**Baths**

- Fill a bath with warm, but not hot, water.
- Add 5–10 drops of essential oil and distribute through the water with your hands.
- Some oils can cause skin irritation in some people so check first by testing in a basin full of water.
- Soak for 5–10 minutes then drain.
- Splash or shower the genital area with cold, or cool, water to stimulate blood flow and drainage.

(*See also* Hydrotherapy and Physiotherapy, page 84.)

**Compresses**

- Fill a bowl with very hot water and add 5–10 drops of essential oil.
- Dip a towel or piece of cloth in the water, wring it out firmly and then wrap it tightly round your abdomen.
- Cover it with a dry towel and retire to bed.
- Rest until the compress cools, or dries out, and then either repeat the procedure or alternate with a cold compress (prepared in the same way as above but using ice cold water).
- The compress helps to relieve pain and reduce inflammation and improves circulation and drainage in the pelvic area. (*See also* naturopathy, pages 82–3.)

**Massage**

- Add 15–20 drops of essential oil to 25ml of a base oil such as pure almond oil.
- Apply some oil to the hands and rub them lightly together to warm the oil.
- Massage gently into the abdomen *in clockwise* movements.
- Cover the body to keep warm and rest while the oil is absorbed through the skin into the bloodstream.

## Clinical ecology (allergy testing)

Clinical ecology looks at the effect of environmental agents, that is the things we eat, drink, breathe, or touch, on our health. Some people develop sensitivities to certain foods, airborne particles, chemicals, etc, and coming into contact with them can produce severe reactions.

Allergy testing involves trying to determine which things produce symptoms in a given individual and then eliminating these from the diet, home, etc. If the body is subsequently strengthened it may be possible to reintroduce certain items at a later date without producing a reaction, but this is very individual.

Allergies have long been thought to play a role in cystitis. It could be that certain foods or drinks, such as orange juice, wheat, tomatoes, tea or coffee, carried in the blood and/or urine cause irritation to the lining of the bladder. Alternatively, if you have had any courses of antibiotics you may have developed a problem with *candida*, a proliferation of 'unfriendly' micro-organisms in the gut (*see* candida pages 67–9). Certain foods, especially sugars and fermented and yeasty foods, encourage the spread of *candida* and make it more likely for you to develop thrush and for bacteria to travel from the anus or vaginal passage into the urethra, ultimately triggering cystitis.

Either allergies can be tested by qualified clinical ecologists using skin tests or electrodermal measuring devices such as the German VEGA machine, or you can determine them for yourself using a process of elimination. However this can take time and requires concentrated effort and will power. If you are really serious about identifying potential allergens and eliminating them it is probably best to consult a professional. If you cannot find one in your area you could try the elimination diet procedure described below.

**Elimination diet**

- Write down everything you eat and drink for one week. Carry a pen and notebook with you everywhere and write things down as you consume them. Do not guess or try to remember what you have had at the end of the day. For this to work it has to be completely accurate.
- Remember to include any seasonings, snacks, tablets, vitamins, water, alcohol and chewing gum as these can also produce reactions in certain individuals. For example, some of the new bottled waters with flavourings contain additives that can irritate.
- In a parallel column in your notebook list any symptoms as they occur. For example if you suddenly feel tired or depressed after a meal note it down. If urination becomes uncomfortable at a certain time of day note that too, and so on.
- At the end of the week sit down, take a long look at the charts and answer the following questions for yourself.
    - Are there any foods that you eat very frequently and miss if you cannot have them, e.g. bread, cheese, sweets?
    - Is your food intake balanced? Do you have fresh fruit and vegetables regularly or do you survive on packaged food? Do you minimize fats and have a good intake of fibre? Do you have a balance of proteins, carbohydrates and other foods?
    - Do you drink plenty of fresh water? Are you consuming large amounts of tea, coffee and/or carbonated drinks?
    - Is there any pattern to your symptoms, for example, always feeling fatigued in the afternoons or always having urinary discomfort after a night out involving alcohol? Does the pattern link to the intake of particular food or drink?
- If certain foods or drinks appear very frequently in your chart and/or appear to be linked to your symptoms, cut them out *completely* from your diet for a period of one month.

* Check labels on food and beware of hidden ingredients such as sugar in bread and mayonnaise.
* Use safe substitutes. For example replace tea with water or mild herbal teas rather than coffee.
* If a lot of items appear to be linked to your symptoms try cutting them out one at a time or eliminating one additional item every week.
* Be prepared for a worsening of symptoms initially as the body detoxifies. Be encouraged that this is usually a sign that you have correctly identified an allergen. Drink plenty of fresh or filtered water and within a day or so symptoms should subside.

- Keep a note of your symptoms during the elimination period. If you see a clear improvement stay off the food/drink for a further eight weeks and then try reintroducing the foods gradually one at a time for a week. Any that trigger symptoms are best avoided indefinitely.

If you suspect *candida* may be your problem you could consult your family doctor or a nutritional therapist specializing in *candida* or try following an anti-candida diet. This basically involves eliminating all foods and drinks that encourage the *candida* organism to thrive and multiply. At the same time as suggesting such a diet, some practitioners prescribe anti-fungals and probiotics such as *Lactobacillus acidophilus* and *Bifidobacterium bifidus* which help to repopulate the gut with 'friendly' bacteria.

**Common symptoms of candida**

- Bloated abdomen
- Alternating diarrhoea and constipation
- Flatulence
- Persistent thrush and/or cystitis
- Menstrual problems
- Fatigue and muscle aching
- Loss of libido

**Anti-candida diet**

Eliminate all the following foods from your diet for at least one month.

- All foods containing yeast, including bread, biscuits, cakes. Substitute rye crackers or 100 per cent rye bread.
- All fermented foods such as vinegar, soy sauce and pickled foods. Make salad dressings with freshly-squeezed lemon juice instead.
- All forms of sugar and sugar products, including sweets, chocolates, honey, maple syrup, sweetened drinks, sweetened yoghurts, etc.
- Milk and dairy products. Use soya products instead.
- All refined white flour products. Use brown flour and whole grains instead.
- All mouldy foods, including mushrooms and old food. Prepare fresh food whenever possible.
- Alcohol, tea and coffee. Use herbal teas and mineral water instead.
- Foods with artificial sweeteners, colourings, preservatives and additives. Eat unadulterated, fresh foods instead.

Include the following foods in your diet.

- Plenty of fresh vegetables, salads and whole grains.
- Garlic, crushed or finely sliced on salads or vegetables.
- Extra virgin, cold pressed olive oil should be the only oil you use.
- Moderate your intake of fruit. Have none for the first week or so (because of their high sugar content) and then reintroduce them gradually. Limit yourself to two fruits per day and avoid very sweet and citrus fruits.

Do not underestimate the importance of allergies and *candida*. A lengthy and detailed case history in Dr Patrick Kingsley's book, *Conquering Cystitis** shows what a devastating effect they can have on a person's life. He describes how Ann, a 33-year-old housewife, had mild symptoms which eventually became so severe that she ended up having shock treatment in a psychiatric hospital – all because of undiagnosed food allergies. A summary of her story is given below.

* Dr. Kingsley's excellent book is now out of print but copies may be obtained direct from 72 Main Street, Osgathorpe, LE12 9TA, UK, priced £7.95 including postage and packaging. The book focuses on diet and nutrition, and details procedures for eliminating allergens and candida.

**Ann's experience with food allergies**

Ann was happily married with two children when she began to suffer from depression, low energy, and crying that would come on for no known reason. Over time the severity and frequency of these 'attacks' worsened and she also developed severe headaches and loss of libido. She felt constantly unwell and her relationships with her husband and children were suffering.

She saw her family doctor several times over the years and he tried various tests but the results were always negative. He also gave her various prescriptions, including tranquillizers, but they only made her worse. Eventually she was referred to a psychiatrist who gave her antidepressants. This time she got even worse. The psychiatrist then admitted her to hospital for 'observation' and it was decided to give her a course of ECT (electroconvulsive shock therapy).

For a time she felt a little better mentally but she also suffered memory loss and had two attacks of cystitis. After a few months her depression and lethargy returned and a further course of ECT was suggested. This time it did not help so much and her memory loss was even worse so she refused the offer of an extended course.

Subsequently she had tonsillitis which was treated with antibiotics. Her throat improved but she developed thrush and, a few days later, cystitis. The cystitis cleared and her doctor gave her pessaries for the thrush. Over the next few months she continued to feel unwell, suffered from digestive problems and had several more bouts of cystitis.

By chance Ann's mother saw an article in a magazine about food allergies and, after reading some books on the subject, Ann and her husband consulted a clinical ecologist. His questioning revealed evidence that she had suffered from food allergies since infancy and that cystitis was just one of a long line of symptoms that had resulted.

The specialist showed her how her different symptoms were linked to food allergies and helped her to identify and eliminate the allergens, change her diet and improve her nutritional status. With his treatment she completely eliminated her cystitis and her general health improved markedly.

Practitioners of Applied Kinesiology (muscle testing) and Radionics also test for allergies but their results are often variable.

**Summary:** Very important in the understanding and prevention of cystitis.

**Healing**

Healing has been practised since ancient times and is widespread amongst lay people, religious institutions, trained healers and other therapists. Basically it involves one or more people healing a person without the use of any instruments or medication.

The most common methods utilized are the laying on of hands and prayer. Not all healers require faith however. The well-known British healer, Matthew Manning, proudly proclaims that he 'takes the faith out of healing' and has demonstrated in laboratory experiments that he can influence cells in a laboratory dish using his hands and mental intention alone.

Other healers invoke a higher power or deity to facilitate healing. Some may also do absent healing by thinking of the person that is sick and then 'sending' them healing from a distance.

Nobody knows exactly how healing works but there is no doubt that in some cases there have been remarkable cures. A report by the British Medical Association in 1956 concluded that 'through spiritual healing recoveries take place that cannot be explained by medical science' and many healers, such as the late Harry Edwards, have claimed 70–80 per cent of their patients show an improvement in their symptoms after healing.

Some argue that this is merely a placebo effect due to the care and attention given by the healers but other investigators have suggested that actual physical changes in the body are produced. Whatever the explanation, the popularity of healing continues unabated and some people with cystitis have tried it. Some report no effect while others say it helped them relax and seemed to help prevent attacks.

***What does healing involve?***

Usually you are asked to relax in either a seated or lying position, fully clothed. Healers then place their hands above or on the body, sometimes holding them still and sometimes moving them to different parts of the body. A few healers, the so-called 'psychic' healers, may actually penetrate the body with their hands or an instrument, such as a knife, but this is rare.

While healing the healer is often quiet or silent as they concentrates on directing healing energies onto the affected part of the body. The person receiving healing often reports feeling sensations of warmth or tingling and often feels very relaxed, or even tired, after the treatment.

Some healing seems to take place instantly while at other times the person returns many times for further healing.

Healers can be contacted through reputable organizations such as the National Federation of Spiritual Healers in the UK, or the American Spiritual Healers Federation or by word of mouth. These organizations have thousands of members and many now work closely with medical doctors and are bound by a code of ethics and conduct.

Healers are not allowed to diagnose but if you go to them with a known condition such as cystitis, diagnosed by your doctor, they will do their best to help. Many offer their services free so be wary of anyone that asks for large sums of money.

Healing is unlikely to cure cystitis, or to be effective in the case of acute infection, but it may help with stress reduction and with strengthening the affected organs.

**Summary:** Healing may be useful for stress-related cystitis. It aids relaxation and may help strengthen internal organs.

## Herbal medicine

Herbal medicine is the oldest known system of medicine and consists of taking the leaves, flowers, bark or other parts of plants, trees or fungi, and taking them internally or externally to prevent or heal disease. In many parts of the world herbal medicine is still one of the dominant forms of medicine and many commonly used drugs in Western medicine, such as aspirin, are based on plant derivatives.

Some herbs can be taken in their raw form and chewed, they can be made into teas or applied in poultices. Alternatively, they can be freeze-dried into powder form, distilled into liquid tinctures or made into ointments. They may be eaten, drunk, applied to the skin, inhaled, added to bath water or used internally in douches or as suppositories.

Some herbs have very mild effects but other can be very toxic, or even poisonous, if taken incorrectly. For this reason it is always important to:

- obtain the best quality herbs from reliable suppliers
- make sure you are fully informed about a herb and how to take it before using it
- consult a trained herbalist for specialist advice
- be very cautious if you are pregnant. Some herbs can be very helpful in pregnancy, during labour and for healing after the birth but others are dangerous. Always get professional advice first.

There are many types of herbalism. The commonest in Western countries are Western medical herbalism and Chinese or Japanese herbal medicine, but there are also Tibetan, Indian, African, Aboriginal and Romany systems of herbal medicine, to name but a few. All herbalists aim to treat the whole person and not just the disease but they may differ in the number and form of the herbs prescribed. Western medical herbalists often use single herbs natural to their locality. Oriental medical herbalists tend to use herbs obtained from the Far East and often favour herbal combinations. Those trained in Chinese herbal medicine sometimes prefer raw herbs and use them in conjunction with acupuncture. Kanpo specialists, trained in Japanese herbal medicine, tend to use smaller dosages and more refined products, such as powders, in preference to raw herbs.

**Herbal medicine for cystitis**

**Parsley** (*Petroselinum sativum*) Chop roughly, infuse in hot water for five minutes then drink. Parsley root and seed can also be taken as a tincture, 5 to 15 drops three to four times per day. Parsley's diuretic action aids urination.

**Cranberry** Drink 250ml of cranberry juice twice every day but avoid highly sweetened products. Do not drink more than one litre a day as this can lead to the formation of kidney stones. If you don't like the taste, or prefer a supplement, you can now get concentrated cranberry extract in tablet form.

Cranberry slightly acidifies the urine, increases urine flow and helps prevent bacteria adhering to the mucous membrane walls in the bladder and urethra.

**Bearberry** *(Uva Ursi)* Take one or two teaspoons of dried leaves infused in water three times a day. Alternatively you can take 250–500mg in tablet form three times a day or 20 to 30 drops of liquid tincture four to six times a day.

Scientific studies have shown that bearberry (upland cranberry) is naturally antiseptic, diuretic and effective against *E. coli* bacteria, but it can be toxic if taken in too high a dosage. Always follow recommended dosages exactly.

**Golden seal** (*Hydrastis canadensis*) Take one to two grams of dried root (500–1000mg if it is freeze-dried) three times a day in a little water. Alternatively take 250–500mg in tablet form three times a day or one teaspoon of a liquid tincture three times daily.

Golden seal is widely used by both herbalists and naturopaths and many scientific studies have demonstrated its effectiveness against a wide range of bacteria including *E. coli.*

**Marshmallow root** (*Althaea officinalis*) Take 10 to 30 grams of powder in warm water three to four times per day.

Marshmallow root reduces inflammation of the mucous membranes and has diuretic properties.

**Buchu** (*Barosma betulina*) Take 10 to 15 drops of liquid tincture three to four times per day.

Buchu is diuretic and antiseptic and a urinary tonic.

**Couch grass** (*Agropyron repens*) Take 5 to 20 drops of liquid tincture three to four times per day.

Couch grass reduces inflammation of the mucous membranes and has diuretic properties.

**Juniper berries** (*Juniperus communis*) Infuse a small handful of berries in water and soak for five minutes. Drain and drink liquid. *Note*: not to be used if pregnant or suffering from kidney disease.

Juniper has strong diuretic effects.

**Saw palmetto berries**, **dandelion root**, **cleavers** (*Galium aperine*) and **nettles** may also be used. Young nettle leaves nipped off the top of wild nettles in the spring (wear gloves to avoid stings from the older leaves further down the stalks!) infused in hot water and then drunk as fresh nettle tea are an excellent kidney tonic.

If using any of these herbs as teas do not add sweeteners or milk. Cammomile tea is also soothing. Some herbs such as **golden seal**, **calendula** and **tea tree** are available in the form of vaginal pessaries and can help to control thrush and reduce the levels of bacteria in the vagina.

*Note:* Cranberry juice is available from any health food shop and many supermarkets. Cranberry extract tablets are available from health food shops and nutritional supplement suppliers. The herbs are available from herbal medicine suppliers, herbalists and naturopaths. High-quality tea tree oil pessaries, which are very effective against thrush, are available from Sandra Beauty (Australian tea tree stockist), 55 Oakleigh Avenue, Whetstone, London N20, UK, tel. 0181 445 6252.

Many Western herbalists now undergo lengthy, professional training. In more rural countries the knowledge of herbal medicine is often passed down in families over many generations as specialist skill is developed.

Certain herbs have long been regarded as beneficial for urinary problems (*see* box below). Many of these can now be obtained 'over the counter' in the form of teas or tinctures while others can simply be picked from the garden and made into infusions or added to food.

Several of the herbs held to improve urinary function, especially cranberry, have been subjected to rigorous scientific investigation and come out well. One study

**Justine's experience with Chinese herbs**

Justine, an unemployed seamstress in her mid-30s, had been suffering from recurrent cystitis when she consulted a practitioner of Chinese herbal medicine. On examination, her tongue was observed to be cracked and dry and red in colour and her pulse was very rapid, especially in the liver position. The practitioner diagnosed a problem of heat and damp in the body and stagnation of liver function. This was partly emotionally generated (she was tense and irritable) and partly due to her excessive consumption of cannabis which, according to Oriental medicine, stagnates liver chi (vital energy).

Justine was given a prescription for the Chinese herbal formula Ba Zheng San (Eight Rectification Powder), a concentrated powder which she had to take daily for some weeks. She was also given some acupuncture treatment to enhance the effect of the herbs.

Gradually Justine became emotionally happier and decreased the amount of cannabis she was taking.

She began to feel physically stronger and, when followed up over two years, had had no further attacks of cystitis. She reported that the treatment had made a 'big difference' to her life.

**Practitioner's comments**: Herbal treatment can help in cystitis but lifestyle change is crucial too. Every case is individual and needs to be managed carefully. Herbs that are cooling or diuretic tend to be used mainly when cystitis is acute. It is also vital to treat the underlying cause which may be deficiency of the kidneys but could also be a weakness of the spleen (causing damp) or the liver (causing heat). Once the infection is cleared you need to build up the person constitutionally to prevent re-infection. Lifestyle factors such as diet and stress levels also need to be considered.

**Chinese herbal formulas**

The following formulas are commonly used for cystitis.

**Zhu Ling Tang** (Polyporous Combination) which helps to drain damp.

**Ba Zheng San** (Eight Rectification Powder) which clears heat.

**Wu Lin San** (Five Ingredient Powder) which clears heat and supports chi and blood.

These formulas can only be obtained on prescription from a Chinese Herbal practitioner.

The East West Herb Shop at 2, Neal's Yard, Covent Garden, London WC2H 9DP has resident practitioners who can advise you.

published in the *Journal of the American Medical Association* in 1994 reported that 300ml of cranberry juice a day led to a significant decrease in the level of bacteria and pus in the urine of a sample of elderly women. Another study in 1968 showed that 73 per cent of subjects with active urinary tract infections (44 females and 16 males) improved when given 16 ounces of cranberry juice daily while 61 per cent of those that improved suffered recurrent infection when the cranberry was withdrawn.

Recent media reports have been concerned with the safety of Chinese medical herbs and their possible toxicity. As a result some herbalists now use blood tests to monitor patients' liver and kidney function. However a study of more than 1000 patients taking Chinese herbs at Great Ormond Street Hospital and another of 48 patients taking Kanpo (Japanese herbal medicine) formulas at the Cavendish Health Centre in London showed no adverse effects. The key seems to be the following of safety guidelines issued by the professional associations. (For further information on safety guidelines for Chinese herbs contact The Register of Chinese Herbal Medicine or the Kanpo Association – *see* Useful Organizations at the end of the book.

**Summary:** Herbal medicine has been shown to be both safe and effective in the prevention and treatment of urinary infections.

### Homeopathy

Homeopathy is a system of medicine based on the principles of 'like cures like' and the minimum dose. These concepts were known to the Greeks in the 5th century BC but were developed into a system of medicine in the 19th century by Samuel Hahnemann, a physician from

Leipzig. He discovered that an illness can be cured if treated with a substance that would normally produce the same symptoms if taken by an otherwise healthy person. Hahnemann also found that the smaller the dose the more potent it could be.

Homoeopathic remedies are made by a process of serial grinding, known as trituration, or serial dilution and shaking, known as succussion. In these processes there is gradually less and less of the original substance present. Yet it seems that an energetic imprint remains that is somehow picked up by the body. Many have been sceptical of this process and there was a furore among the scientific community when the French scientist Jean Bienveniste claimed to have demonstrated it under laboratory conditions. Yet there can be little doubt that homeopathy is effective. It is practised throughout the world, is especially popular in Europe and India and is used by many medical doctors.

In homeopathy the aim is to stimulate the body's response to illness rather than suppress it. For this reason symptoms may initially get worse before they get better as the body's healing defences are mobilized.

Homeopathic remedies can be taken in the form of tablets or pillules or in liquid tinctures preserved in alcohol. If you are allergic to dairy products make sure that the tablets/pills are lactose free and, if sensitive to alcohol, place the tincture drops in a little warm water and let the alcohol evaporate. For babies and toddlers homoeopathic sugar granules which simply dissolve on the tongue can be used.

For cystitis the homoeopathic remedy is selected on the basis of individual symptoms (*see* box). It is always advisable to consult a professional homoeopath for advice but in many countries the remedies are bought over the counter for home use as they are so safe, effective and inexpensive.

**Homoeopathic remedies for cystitis**

The remedies listed below can help alleviate immediate symptoms. Read through the list and carefully select the description that most closely resembles your current condition. Take only one remedy at a time and keep to the potency listed (the numbers 6c and 30c refer to the potency of the remedy, that is, the number of times the tincture of the substance has been diluted and shaken, or succussed. In homeopathy the more times a substance is diluted the more potent it is thought to become).

Take the appropriate remedy every half an hour for up to ten doses to relieve urinary discomfort. Tablets or pills may be dissolved on the tongue or chewed. Tinctures can be added to half a wine glass of water. Avoid all tea, coffee and mint (including mint toothpaste) while taking the remedy and allow 30 minutes before or after consuming food or drink or smoking.

It is vital that you *stop* taking the remedy as soon as you have a marked improvement and only take more if symptoms recur. If you see no change after six doses stop and check the chart again for a more suitable remedy or seek professional advice. Consult a trained homoeopath for constitutional treatment to help prevent recurring cystitis.

**Cantharis 30c** Burning, cutting pains in lower abdomen too severe to ignore; non-stop urge to urinate; ache in small of back tends to get worse in afternoon; merest trickle of urine with blood in it; inability to empty bladder properly.
**Nux 6c** Frequent and painful urging with little result.
**Apis 30c** Sharp, stinging pains in lower abdomen; frequent urge to urinate; urine scanty, hot, and bloody; symptoms seem worse for heat and better for cold.
**Belladonna 30c** Burning sensation along urethra; bladder sensitive to jarring; urine bright red with little clots of blood in it; urging persists even after urine has been passed.
**Tarentula 6c** High fever; excruciating pain in bladder area; bladder swollen and hard; feeling extremely restless; great sense of hurry.

**Berberis 6c** Urine slimy, with fine mucus in it; burning, radiating pains which get worse during and after passing urine, and during rest.
**Causticum 6c** Frequent urge to pass urine, made worse by coughing and sneezing; acute sensitivity to cold; obeying urge produces nothing but is followed, 15 minutes later, by involuntary passage of urine; itching around urethral opening, perhaps with vaginal discharge.
**Dulcamara 6c** Attack comes on after getting damp and cold after exertion, especially in autumn; urine bloody and frequent.
**Sarsaparilla 6c** Pains come on as urination ceases; urine thick and milky-looking; urgency and pressure to pass urine; feeling thirsty.
**Terebinth 6c** Frequency and burning sensation as urine is passed, with pain in small of back; blood in urine; drowsiness; tingling in ears; tongue red and shiny; rest makes symptoms worse but walking in open air alleviates them.
**Staphisagria 6c** Attack comes on after sexual intercourse or after catheterization for an operation; urethra feels as if a drop of urine is continuously trickling along it; burning sensation almost constant, even when not passing water.
**Clematis 6c** Stream of urine slow and intermittent.
**Arsenicum 6c** Burning pains in lower abdomen; feeling restless, chilly, and anxious.
**Camphora 6c** Pain worse at start of urination; no urine passed despite intense and urgent straining; muscles at base of bladder in spasm; cold makes symptoms worse.

Excerpted from *The Family Guide to Homeopathy* by Dr Andrew Lockie (Hamish Hamilton 1989) and reprinted with kind permission from Dr Andrew Lockie and Penguin Books.

**Summary:** Homeopathy can help relieve acute symptoms and constitutional treatment may help prevent recurrent cystitis.

## Massage

There are many forms of therapeutic massage. Most help to relieve muscle tension, promote relaxation and increase the circulation of blood and lymph. All of these can be beneficial to a cystitis sufferer seeking to prevent attacks and improve his or her general health. Shiatsu, a form of Japanese massage which works on the meridian system (*see* Acupuncture section, page 53–7), may also help to improve bladder and kidney function.

## Naturopathy

Naturopaths try to mobilize the natural healing forces of the body by rectifying chemical, mechanical and/or psychological imbalances. They place a lot of importance on diet, may recommend fasting and detoxification regimes including hydrotherapy and often use homoeopathic and herbal remedies and osteopathic techniques. (*See* Herbal Medicine, page 72–78, Homeopathy, page 78–81 and Osteopathy, page 85–88.) The John Bastyr College in the USA has done extensive research demonstrating its effectiveness for both acute and chronic diseases.

A naturopath treating someone prone to cystitis will want to ensure that the person has good digestion and elimination, a balanced diet and no spinal imbalance or lesion that could cause degradation of the tissues of the urogenital organs. A typical naturopathic purification regime is given opposite. It can be useful for both chronic and acute cystitis but is best followed under the guidance of a qualified practitioner.

**Naturopathic treatment for cystitis**

**1 Diet to purify kidneys, bladder and urethra.**

*Stage 1: Liquid fast*

For five to seven days take no solids and drink the following daily.

- Parsley tea (diuretic action) – as much as you like.
- Watermelon seed tea (purifies) – according to thirst.
- Cranberry juice (unsweetened) (slightly acidifies urine, increases urine flow, and prevents bacteria adhering to the mucous membrane walls of bladder and urethra) – up to 250ml twice a day.
- Apple cider vinegar, water, and pure honey (one cup three times per day).

*Stage 2: Reintroduction of solids*

For seven to ten days, or until condition clears; eat and drink according to the following regime.

- Continue to drink eight or more glasses of the liquids listed above (i.e. no tea, coffee, alcohol, carbonated drinks). Freshly made vegetable juices can be added.
- Avoid all dairy and animal produce, including eggs. Stick to vegetarian foods.
- Eat plenty of the following:
  - fresh vegetables steamed or simmered; asparagus, celery, parsnips and carrots are especially good
  - whole grains
  - salads including parsley and watercress
  - baked potatoes
  - pulses especially kidney and aduki beans; soak overnight, rinse well and simmer slowly removing the scum as they cook and draining before eating
  - watermelon and non-citrus fruits (avoid citrus fruits)
- condiments: avoid salt, use garlic for flavour

After this reintroduce other foods gradually. Continue to avoid large amounts of animal protein as this overtaxes the kidneys.

### 2 Hydrotherapy and physiotherapy

Hot sitz-baths can be used to improve pelvic circulation and relieve pain. They can be used in acute cystitis or once or twice a week to prevent cystitis.

- Warm the room and wrap your upper body in towels.
- Fill the bath half full with water at 37–38 degrees centigrade (98–99 degrees Farenheit). Use a water thermometer for the temperature should be exact. Herbs or aromatherapy oils could be added (*see* Aromatherapy, pages 61–4 and Herbal Medicine, pages 74–5).
- Immerse your buttocks and hips only in the water. Keep the top half of your body wrapped and warm.
- Remain in the bath for 30 minutes, topping up with hot water occasionally to keep the temperature constant.

Hot and cold compresses can be used to improve circulation and drainage in the pelvic region. (*See* also Aromatherapy, pages 61–3.)

### 3 Elimination

Use gentle enemas, naturally laxative foods and plenty of dietary fibre to regulate bowel function and encourage the elimination of toxins.

### 4 Nutrition

Ensure good nutritional balance using supplements and probiotics as necessary (*see* Candida, pages 67–8 and Diet and Nutrition, page 100)

**Edna's story**

Edna, a 75-year-old pensioner, visited a naturopath complaining of mild incontinence, smelly urine and some discomfort on urinating. She had had several cystitis attacks over the years which she had either cleared herself 'by drinking lots of water' or, in severe cases, had treated with antibiotics. She wondered if her urinary weakness was due to 'old age'.

The naturopath gave Edna a herbal preparation for strengthening the bladder (containing Uva Ursi) and one for boosting immunity (containing Echinacea). He suggested changes to her diet and recommended four small glasses of cranberry juice daily in place of tea and coffee. He also prescribed her a course of probiotics (*see* pages 30, 67 and 102) as examination suggested that she had mild thrush which was producing a smelly discharge.

After four weeks of following this regime Edna returned with a beaming smile. 'My waterworks are back to normal and I've even been able to take up bowls again!'

**Summary:** Naturopathy can help relieve chronic and acute cystitis by mobilizing the body's natural healing mechanisms.

## Osteopathy and Chiropractic

The manipulative therapies of osteopathy and chiropractic are probably the most widely accepted forms of natural therapy within orthodox medicine today. The USA, Australia, New Zealand, and most European countries legally recognize practitioners, and standards of training are high.

Osteopathy as it exists today dates back to the end of the 19th century and the work of Dr Andrew Still, who studied engineering and became interested in the effects of mechanical malfunction of the skeletal system on the body systems and internal organs. The system of chiropractic was formalized by a Canadian, Dr David Palmer, at around the same time.

Both therapies involve manipulation of the spine and joints by hand in order to restore normal health and function. Chiropractic tends to be more vigorous than osteopathy and have more reliance on X-rays while osteopathy often incorporates soft tissue massage. Some osteopaths use the even subtler techniques of cranial osteopathy which manipulates the energy patterns of the body by balancing the flow of cerebrospinal fluid in the cranium.

Although manipulative therapies are generally associated with joint problems and bad backs, it has long been known that altering the mechanics of the body can also improve the functioning of the internal organs as well as the circulation of blood and fluids. The growing body of research in the field supports this.

People who suffer from cystitis often have a tendency for congestion in the pelvic region which inhibits the nerve supply and the flow of blood and lymph to and from the bladder and kidneys. This may be due to scarring from repeated infections, to falls and injuries which affect pelvic balance, to poor posture, or to problems associated with childbirth. If muscle tone and pelvic floor muscles are weakened after giving birth, or if the pelvis tips and the positioning of the pelvic organs is imbalanced, there is more likelihood of cystitis occurring.

In such cases manipulative therapies can help to reposition the pelvic organs and improve circulation in the surrounding tissues, thereby helping to prevent recurrent cystitis. A small number of osteopaths are also able to work internally to correct the positioning of the pelvic organs.

Manipulative treatment should always be carried out by a qualified professional and may include advice on diet, hygiene and lifestyle and preventive exercises too.

**Ruth's story**

Ruth, a professional woman in her forties, developed cystitis for the first time when resuming love-making after childbirth. She had had a long labour and a difficult birth that ended in a forceps delivery and had felt sore and uncomfortable for weeks afterwards. The cystitis had cleared after a course of antibiotics but had returned a few months later. A further course of antibiotics had helped but she was fearful of having cystitis again.

Ruth visited an osteopath because of some back pain she had been having and was surprised when the osteopath, after taking her history, said that the back pain and cystitis problems might be connected to her childbirth. She had not connected the two and had had no idea that osteopathy might help prevent cystitis.

The osteopath examined her spine and pelvis and found strong compression in her sacrum, restricted movement in the pelvic joints and poor muscle tone. It was as if everything had 'seized up' in that area of Ruth's body. Ruth admitted to having been very frightened and tense during the birth and said that her periods, which had returned recently, were more uncomfortable than before.

The osteopath gave Ruth five treatments in which she used gentle soft tissue massage and manipulative techniques combined with some cranio-sacral therapy. She also gave her advice on hygiene procedures and on the use of lubricants during intercourse. Over the course of the treatments Ruth started to feel more mobile in her lower body and her back pain disappeared. She found she was sleeping better and her periods normalized too. Six months later she had had no further bouts of cystitis and was planning to try for a second baby later in the year. This time she planned to have osteopathy during her pregnancy and after the birth too.

**Summary**: Osteopathy and chiropractic can help alleviate and prevent cystitis in cases where there is congestion and imbalance in the pelvic organs. These may also prevent the need for surgery.

### Reflexology

Reflexology dates back to ancient Egypt and involves the application of fingertip pressure to reflex points on the feet to mobilize the body's natural healing ability and improve internal organ function.

Anyone can practise reflexology and it is popular among massage therapists and beauticians. Although it is safe to practise oneself it is best to consult an experienced practitioner as too strong a pressure in the wrong places can cause excessive detoxification leading to discomfort. It is also much more relaxing to lie down and have it done to you, which probably enhances its benefits.

Massage of the kidney, bladder and urinary reflex points will stimulate bladder function and help improve water metabolism in the body.

**Gentle massage with the tip of the thumb on these reflex points stimulates urinary function.**

**1 The kidney reflexes (both feet)**

**2 The bladder, ureter and urethra reflexes (both feet)**

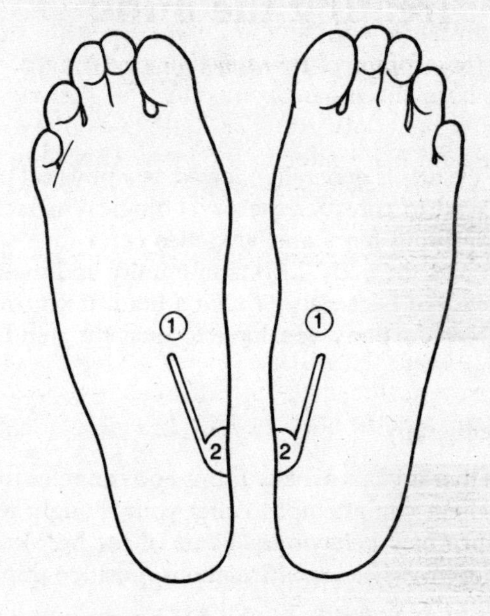


**Fig. 4 Reflex points for the urinary system**

Metamorphic Technique, developed by naturopath and reflexologist Robert St John in the 1960s, is a specialized form of reflexology that concentrates on the spinal reflexes in the foot. It too seems to promote relaxation and healing and may be of help to those prone to cystitis.

**Summary:** Reflexology promotes relaxation and may stimulate urinary function. It is probably most useful in the prevention of cystitis.

CHAPTER 8

# Treating the mind

*Psychological therapies for cystitis*

Although cystitis is generally viewed as a physical problem it is vital to consider the psychological aspects as well. Underlying fears and anxieties can cause stress which fatigues the body, lowers immunity and makes it more likely that bacteria will take a hold. If you really want to treat the body you have to treat the mind and emotions as well.

## Cognitive therapy

Cognitive therapy takes many forms and can refer to any therapy where you attempt to alter your thought forms and produce new behaviours. Some of the best-known cognitive approaches are affirmations, positive thinking and visualizations.

### *Affirmations*

Affirmations are a way of using positive thoughts to promote wellbeing. They are mental messages which can guide the body towards wellness and harmony of mind, body and spirit. Probably the best-known affirmations are those created by Louise Hay in her best-seller, *You Can Heal Your Life* (Eden Grove, USA, 1988).

Hay argues that every disease is linked to a particular type of mental pattern. Bladder and kidney problems, she suggests, are linked to feelings of anxiety, disappointment and shame, a fear of letting go, a desire to hold on to old ideas, and a critical nature, or fear of being criticized. The affirmations to dispel such feeling are 'I comfortably and easily release the old and welcome the new in my life. I am safe' and 'Divine right action is always taking place in my life. Only good comes from each experience. It is safe to grow up'.

It may be hard at first to convince yourself of the power of affirmations or even to say them to yourself! Hay suggests that you say them out loud to yourself while looking in a mirror and then, as you become more confident, start to repeat them silently in your mind. Repeat them as often as possible throughout the day and especially first thing in the morning and last thing at night to programme your mind. Countless people testify that they work.

### *Taoist healing*

Affirmations also have a parallel in Oriental medical healing systems. According to traditional Chinese medicine the kidneys and bladder are linked to the emotion of fear. Fears and anxieties can inhibit the flow of energy within the bladder and kidney meridians and cause stagnation around the internal organs, visualized as a black cloud. To dispel this and promote healing, Taoist healers recommend that you 'put a smile' on the internal organs every day by visualizing them as vibrant and healthy and by talking to them! Modern research has suggested that plants thrive when they are spoken to, so why not one's internal organs? Try waking up every morning and telling your kidneys and bladder that you love them and know they can do a good job throughout the day, and see what happens!

### *Positive thinking*

This involves replacing negative mental statements with positive ones. Any debilitating and painful condition such as cystitis produces negative thoughts such as 'I am never going to get better', 'I can't stand this pain' etc. Often these thoughts are unconscious, destroying our confidence without us even realizing it.

First you need to become aware of your negative thoughts. The next step is to halt them and replace them with a positive statement, either spoken out loud or repeated mentally. For example, the thought 'I am never going to get better' is stopped and replaced with 'Every day I am getting better'.

Repetition of positive mental thoughts sends powerful messages to the brain and can actually affect brain chemicals and the production of hormones. Research has shown that people who are positive in outlook and laugh a lot have quite a different chemical make up to those who feel pessimistic and depressed. One of the differences is in the production of endorphins, the brain's natural opiates and painkillers. High levels of these chemicals may play a role in resistance to disease and the ability of the body to fight infection.

### *Visualization*

Another way that the power of the mind can be harnessed is through creating positive mental images. Everyone uses images in his or her mental processing and these images affect our memory and understanding of events.

Art therapy has revealed that people with diseased or weak organs tend to have a very poor mental image of the affected body part. People with cancer, for example, often draw the affected part of their body in dark colours and heavy lines. Many practitioners, such as the Simontons in America, argue that a positive visual image with colour and light can facilitate healing of the diseased organ. In art therapy it can be seen that as the person feels more positive about his or her health and recovery, colours spontaneously become lighter and drawings have more movement.

Try taking a plain sheet of paper and drawing your bladder and kidneys. Do you know precisely where they are located in the body and how they look, their shape, size, colour, etc?

Look them up in a colour anatomy book if you can and from now on always carry a positive, healthy image of them in your mind.

This positive visualization can help to strengthen kidney and bladder function as it facilitates the release of muscular tension and promotes circulation and the flow of vital energy.

## Counselling and Psychotherapy

Talking through problems can help relieve anxiety and stress and promote relaxation in the body. Sometimes talking to a partner, friend or relative is best but at other times professional help from someone who is detached from the situation is needed. At such times counsellors, psychotherapists and/or psychologists may be of help.

### *Counselling*

Counselling enables you to talk through your problems with someone trained to listen non-judgementally who can support you and help you to explore solutions to problems. A professional counsellor will not tell you what to do but will help you to express your feelings, see your situation more clearly and come to a decision about what action you need to take.

Co-counselling is where you set up a counselling relationship with a friend and give each other specific periods of time just to talk or listen and then feed back what you have heard. This process can help to clarify issues and throw out possible solutions.

### *Psychotherapy*

Psychotherapy involves delving deeper into unconscious processes and childhood experiences that may be the underlying cause of current insecurities or emotional problems. There are many, many different forms of psychotherapy. Some are brief while many involve sessions over long periods. Some involve working with the unconscious and dreams while others are more analytic. Find out everything you can about the therapy before making a choice.

### *Psychology*

Clinical psychologists are trained in non-drug approaches to behavioural and emotional problems. They can help you to understand the causes of your anxieties and fears and suggest techniques to enable you to change them.

**Amy's story**

Amy, a shy eight-year-old, was brought to see a clinical psychologist by her mother because of bed wetting. She had started wetting her bed two months earlier, following the death of her grandmother, to whom she had been very close. Her day-time bladder control had also deteriorated. She had recently lost control while at school and wet herself in the playground. Other children had taunted her and she was reluctant to go to school. On several occasions she had complained of discomfort when going to the toilet and on one occasion the doctor had diagnosed cystitis and prescribed antibiotics.

The psychologist talked with both Amy and her mother. The mother told how Amy was becoming increasingly anxious and withdrawn. Although she wanted to be sympathetic the mother was becoming irritated because of the inconvenience of changing the wet beds all the time. She said that she had been spending less time with Amy because she was preoccupied with her own grief at the death of her mother.

Amy told how upset she had been to lose her grandmother. She now felt afraid that her mother might die too and felt it had been her fault in some way although she knew it wasn't really. She also missed the closeness she had had with both her mum and grandmother and she was scared of the teasing children at school.

The psychologist helped Amy and her mother talk through and share their grief about their bereavement. She showed the mother how much Amy needed her support and enabled them to find new ways to be together once more. Talking through the bereavement helped reduce Amy's anxieties about death and her feelings of guilt. The psychologist also gave Amy some simple exercises to boost her confidence and enabled her to find a new role at school which strengthened friendships and helped her overcome the fear of being teased.

Finally the psychologist taught Amy and her mother measures for controlling urination which included not drinking after a certain time in the evening, waking in the night to empty her bladder, always emptying her bladder promptly and fully during the day and changing underwear immediately after any leakage to prevent the spread of infection.

Within a few weeks Amy became relaxed and happier, her bladder control improved and she had no further infections. The psychologist had helped her and her mother work through a painful life experience and also make changes that boosted Amy's confidence and improved her bladder control.

## Flower remedies

Flower remedies use the essence of plants to treat the negative states of mind that are thought to underlie disease. The best-known in the West are probably the Bach Flower Remedies created by Dr Edward Bach in Oxfordshire earlier this century, but there are also flower remedies from Australia, Africa, the Himalayas and the rain forests, to name but a few. (For a comprehensive guide see Clare Harvey and Amanda Cochrane's excellent book, *The Encyclopaedia of Flower Remedies*, Thorsons, 1995.)

The flower remedies have been described as 'liquid consciousness' that carries the energetic blueprint of the plant and transforms mental patterns. The beauty is that they are safe, inexpensive and non-toxic and can be used at the same time as drugs or other therapies to promote healing.

Flower remedies are always chosen to suit the whole person rather than for any specific symptom, but some of the remedies that may be indicated for a person with cystitis are given below to illustrate the range available. Of course it is always best to consult an experienced practitioner who can select the remedies most suited to you as an individual.

## Hypnotherapy

In hypnotherapy a deep state of relaxation is induced and suggestions are planted in the subconscious mind to influence the mind and body in the waking state. In most medical hypnosis you are fully aware of what is going on but your deep state of relaxation means the mind is very receptive to the planting of ideas. It is really a form of mental programming that bypasses the conscious mind.

**Flower remedies for cystitis**

**Mimulus** (a Bach Flower Remedy first created by Dr Edward Bach and now made by his successors at the Edward Bach Centre in Oxfordshire)
*Action:* For known fears of everyday things like pain, the dark and loneliness. Gives courage and helps overcome fears. **Aspen** may also be indicated for unknown fears and feelings of apprehension and uneasiness. Helps put fears in perspective. **Rescue Remedy** is also helpful.

**Pansy** (a Petit Fleur Essence created by Judy Graham in America)
*Action:* Affects adrenal and kidney function and helps eliminate toxins. Helps overcome deep-seated grief from loss of a loved one.

**Marigold** (a Petit Fleur Essence created by Judy Graham in America)
*Action:* For sexual guilt and confusion. Balances hormones and prostate function and the male and female sides of oneself.

**Fringed Violet** (a Bush Flower Remedy from Australia created by fifth-generation herbalist Ian White)
*Action:* For shock and trauma, drained energy and vitality and poor recuperation. **Bush Iris** and **Dagger Hakea** may also be indicated.

**Brown Kelp** (Canadian Sea Essence created by Sabina Petitt from marine life of the Pacific Northwest)
*Action:* Works on the bladder meridian and helps bladder infections and fluid imbalances. Helps shift perception and lift fear and confusion.

The remedies are taken by putting a few drops of the liquid tinctures in water and sipping them two to four times a day.

Research has shown that hypnosis can help reduce pain, anxiety and tension so it may be useful for cystitis sufferers with a lot of stress and anxiety. Because it is open to abuse it is especially important to consult a trained and reliable therapist.

### Meditation

Meditation induces a state of mental calm and concentration, and can help relieve stress and promote healing. There are many different techniques involving breathing, visualization and the use of *mantras*, sounds or words of power.

Research has shown that in a meditative state the body is relaxed, physiological and mental processes are slowed and healing can take place.

### Relaxation training

Relaxation training helps develop awareness of, and then prevent, the build-up of muscle tension that is part and parcel of modern-day stress. The best-known relaxation training is probably Jacobson's Progressive Relaxation which involves sequentially tensing and then relaxing different muscles in the body. The aim is to learn to feel when a muscle is tense and then develop the ability to release it.

Other techniques, such as Autogenic training, developed by Schultz, use mental commands and visualization to induce a sense of relaxation throughout the body. The key commands are feelings of heaviness, warmth and calm.

When the body is relaxed blood and lymph can circulate freely and immune function is enhanced. Many people who suffer recurrent cystitis are tense and anxious and fearful of the pain that each bout may bring. Relaxation is then an important step in total healing.

## Sexual therapy

Sex is often closely linked to cystitis, and emotional issues can be as important as the physical aspects. If there are relationship problems, or fears and anxieties concerning sex, there will be tension and less production of the natural lubricants that come with sexual arousal. As a result there is increased likelihood of bruising and inflammation leading to infection.

It may be that just talking things through with your partner is sufficient to diffuse tension and create more relaxed close contact. Sometimes, however, sexual fears and guilt or shame, for example in the case of someone who has been abused, are so deep-seated that professional help is required. Frigidity and sexual inadequacy may also be a problem.

A trained counsellor or psychotherapist will be able to help with emotional issues but if the problems are more sexual then a clinical psychologist or trained sex therapist may be better.

CHAPTER 9

# Diet and nutrition

A balanced, healthy diet is crucial to the prevention of cystitis as well as to general health. Modern-day Western diets tend to be laden with junk foods, saturated fats, refined flours and sugars and laced with sweetened, carbonated drinks or stimulant drinks such as tea and coffee. All of these have a ruinous effect on physical health over the years, causing clogging of the arteries and veins, poor absorption of nutrients, deteriorating function of the internal organs and degradation of the tissues. If you are serious about getting well and optimizing your health you must be willing to make some effort with your diet and implement changes.

The key to a healthy diet is plenty of fresh vegetables (preferably organic or home grown for freshness and lack of harmful chemicals and preservatives), whole grains, locally grown fruit, vegetarian protein, essential fatty acids and lots of fresh water, natural juices and mild herbal teas. Cooking is important too with steaming or conservative boiling and simmering being the best way to preserve nutrients.

A healthy daily diet should be predominantly *alkaline* in nature as this provides the best environment for the absorption of nutrients and for intercellular exchange of nutrients and waste products. A typical junk food diet, or one high in animal protein, sugars and refined carbohydrates, is very *acidic* in nature and predisposes the body to poor absorption of nutrients and a build-up of toxins.

**A healthy diet to promote health and prevent cystitis**

- Eat plenty of fresh vegetables, preferably organic and conservatively cooked.
- Always select whole grains (brown rice, whole wheat pasta, muesli, rye bread, etc.) in preference to white, refined products.
- Consume mainly or all vegetable protein. Limit your intake of animal proteins which are harder for the body to digest.
- Use pure, unsaturated oils such as flaxseed to provide essential fatty acids.
- Take moderate amounts of local fruits. Avoid unseasonable, citrus and tropical fruits.
- Avoid or limit all dairy produce, which is very acidic in nature. Vegetables, seaweeds and sesame seeds are also far better sources of calcium and the calcium is more easily absorbed by the body.
- Drink plenty of good quality water, home-made vegetable and fruit juices and mild herbal teas. (Aim for at least 1.5–2 litres fluid per day and more if it's hot or you're exercising.) Eliminate or limit coffee, tea, colas and sweetened, carbonated drinks which all cause bladder irritation and interfere with fluid metabolism.

In certain cases where a person is very run down or not able to prepare an adequate diet, a regimen of nutritional supplements may be helpful. The most vital nutrients are those that boost immune function, maintain the integrity of cells and mucous membranes and promote healing. A typical nutritional regime is given on page 102.

## Nutritional supplements

### Vitamins and minerals

**Vitamin C:** 500mg every two hours or up to six times daily. Bioflavinoid complexes or buffered types, such as magnesium ascorbate, are well tolerated and less detrimental for teeth. If bowels become loose decrease the dose.
Boosts immune function and tissue repair and helps fight infection.

**Vitamin A:** 25,000 iu per day. Do not exceed this dosage without medical supervision. Contraindicated during pregnancy.
Essential for health of the mucous membranes.

**Vitamin B complex:** twice a day. (Yeast-free type is best.)
Strengthens nervous system and aids detoxification.

**Vitamin E:** 400 iu one to two times per day.
Promotes healing of skin tissues.

**Flaxseed oil:** 1000 mg a day.
Essential fatty acid that regulates nervous and other systems.

**Zinc (picolinate):** 30 mg every evening taken *with water only*.
Boosts immune function and tissue repair.

### Other supplements

**Garlic:** take fresh or take one to three capsules a day.
Boosts immunity and resistance to infection.

***Acidophilus Lactobacillus*** and ***Bifidobacterium bifidum:***
Probiotics, available in powder form or capsules. Take first thing in the morning and last thing at night and consume no hot drink within 30 minutes. Get a non-dairy form if you are dairy sensitive.

Buy good quality products from reputable suppliers. Where possible use vegetable capsules rather than gelatine and avoid products with many fillers and preservatives.

**Note**: The amounts quoted above are for *adults*. Nutritional supplements should only be given to children under the guidance of an experienced nutritional therapist. All the above supplements, with the exception of zinc and the probiotics, *must be taken with food.*

CHAPTER 10

# How to find and choose a natural therapist

*Tips and guidelines for finding reliable help*

The number of qualified practitioners of natural therapies is increasing all the time and it is becoming easier to find one that will provide you with reliable help. However, training systems, professional organizations and advertising procedures vary from country to country so it helps to know where to look and what to look for.

## How to find a qualified therapist

Probably the best way to locate a good therapist is by word of mouth. Ask friends, family, neighbours or work colleagues if they can recommend anyone. You could also try asking your family doctor. If he or she is informed about and interested in natural therapies they may be part of the practice or a referral may be possible. A local pharmacist may also have information or you could try calling local natural therapists to ask if they know of anyone practising the therapy you are seeking.

***National sources***

The national professional associations for each therapy maintain up-to-date directories of their members and are usually willing to provide lists of local practitioners and supply information about the therapy. All reputable practitioners are members of one or another professional association. There is also an increasing number of 'umbrella' organizations concerned with natural therapies that can provide information about a range of therapies and lists of practitioners.

National organizations concerned with cystitis or support groups (local and national) may also be able to help (*see* Appendix A). The relevant addresses and phone numbers can usually be obtained from phone companies or libraries.

If you are computer literate you may get good sources on the Internet, or via computer information services, but always check them out thoroughly as you do not always know the source of the information!

***Local sources***

Local natural health centres, health food stores, libraries, alternative book stores, citizens' advice bureaux or neighbourhood centres may hold lists of local practitioners or display advertising cards. However, do be wary of unscrupulous advertisers. Many professional associations forbid private advertising and only allow corporate entries in directories or newspapers, so those advertising prominently may not be the best or the most reputable.

Print is another good source of therapists. Try local community directories, commercial phone directories or even local newspapers and magazines. Sometimes multi-disciplinary clinics advertise their facilities in these sources and you can then call up and ask what therapies are available. Some clinics also offer a screening procedure to help you choose the right therapy for you.

**Ten ways of finding a therapist**

- Word of mouth (one of the best ways)
- Doctor's surgeries or health centres
- National associations of therapists (*see* Appendix A)
- National organizations concerned with cystitis (*see* Appendix A)
- Local or national support groups for cystitis
- Computer networks such as the Internet
- Local natural health centres
- Local health food or alternative book stores
- Public libraries, information centres and advice bureaux
- Local directories, newspapers and magazines

## Selecting a therapist

Once you have located a therapist you need to use your judgement to decide if the person is right for you. Check the following:

- the therapist's qualifications and training
- how long has he been in practice
- whether he belonged to a recognized professional body with an established code of conduct
- whether he has professional indemnity insurance
- what experience he has had in treating cystitis

Most practitioners will be happy to answer your questions. You may also want to check out the practice to see if it is clean and tidy and looks professional.

Make sure you feel comfortable with the therapist. If you don't gel together find another one. Your relationship is as important as the therapy and you need to feel you can trust the person and have confidence in his skills.

### Checking professional associations

Practitioners generally join professional associations after qualifying from a recognized training course. The associations provide a number of services including:

- monitoring education and training
- providing the public with information about their discipline
- maintaining up-to-date directories of members
- arranging indemnity insurance for members
- dealing with complaints and disciplinary procedures
- informing members of legal changes

Reputable associations will provide full information about their aims and activities directly to the public. You could check out their status by asking the following questions.

- When was the association founded?
- How many members does it have?
- How do its members gain admission to its register?
- Does it have a code of conduct, complaints mechanism and disciplinary procedures for its members?
- Do all members have professional indemnity insurance covering accidental damage, negligence and malpractice?
- Is it linked to any particular school or do its members come from more than one training institution? Is it part of a larger network of organizations? Associations with wider links may have higher standards and more credibility.
- Is it a charity, educational trust or a private company? Charities are non-profit-making and exist to promote the therapies and serve the public interest. Private companies are more financially motivated.

## Checking training and qualifications

Don't be afraid to ask what the letters after a therapist's name mean or to ask for details of her training.

- How long is the training?
- Is it full or part time?
- Does it include seeing patients under supervision? You need to be sure that the person has had practical training, not just theoretical.
- Is the qualification recognized? If so, by whom?

As more medical doctors train in natural therapies it is becoming easier to find practitioners who are also medically qualified if this is your preference. However, being medically qualified doesn't necessarily mean that the person is an expert in your chosen therapy. In the UK, for example, a medical doctor can practise acupuncture after just a weekend course of training or just reading an acupuncture book. Such a person's level of expertise can hardly compare with that of someone who has done three years, or more, specialist training in acupuncture. So it is worthwhile enquiring exactly what training the practitioner has had.

## Making the choice

Once you have checked out the therapist's training, qualifications, professional membership and experience with cystitis the next step is to try the treatment. If you feel comfortable with the therapist and happy with the treatment then be willing to give the therapy a fair trial by following the therapist's advice conscientiously and completing a course of treatment. However, if at any stage you are unhappy with the therapist or dissatisfied with the treatment don't be afraid to discontinue the therapy.

*Cautions*

- Check out the costs of treatment and remedies beforehand. Expect to pay the going rate for the treatment and additional amounts for any medicines but be wary of being asked to pay large amounts 'up-front'. Many practitioners offer concessions for children, the elderly and those with financial difficulties, so ask about these if applicable.
- Be wary of any therapist who promises you a 'cure' or who advises you to stop other medications. Only change drug treatment on the advice of your family doctor.
- If you need to undress feel free to have someone of the same sex with you as a chaperone. Should the therapist make any sort of sexual advance to you leave immediately and make a report to the relevant professional association.
- If the practice is a busy one book yourself in for a series of treatments to ensure continuity but always give notice if you need to cancel otherwise you may be charged.

**What to do if things go wrong**

If you feel the therapy is not working you must first ask yourself if you have given it a fair trial. Have you given it enough time to work? (Most natural remedies work more slowly than modern drug treatments and some make you feel worse before you get better.) Have you had sufficient treatment? Have you followed all the advice given by the therapist?

If your dissatisfaction is with the therapist rather than the therapy you must first ask yourself if you feel the therapist has genuinely failed you or if you have had a personality clash and you are simply better off seeking treatment elsewhere. If you are sure the therapist has been incompetent, negligent, unprofessional or unethical you should take action. This will help to clarify the matter, allow the therapist to correct the situation if possible and protect yourself and other future clients if necessary.

- If you can, discuss the matter directly with the therapist. This will enable him or her to put things right if there has been a genuine misunderstanding.
- If you are unable to discuss the matter with the therapist, or you are dissatisfied with the response you got, inform the professional association to which your therapist belongs or the management if you received treatment in a health centre. This should ensure independent investigation of the problem and disciplinary procedures if appropriate.
- If the offence committed is a criminal one report it to the police or see a lawyer or citizen's advice bureau for advice.
- If you have a genuine grievance tell others about your experience so that they may be warned. Bad publicity damages practitioners' reputations and can quickly put them out of business. However, never spread malicious, unfounded gossip or you could find yourself at risk of legal action from the practitioner.

## Summary

Most therapists are caring, responsible individuals who have invested considerable time, money and effort in training in their chosen therapy or therapies. The majority are highly professional and genuinely concerned to assist you in your healing. However, there are always exceptions in every profession and you should be on the look out for those who are incompetent or fraudulent.

Taking responsibility for your own health is the key

to getting the best from any given therapy. Use your own judgement and intuition to select an appropriate therapy and therapist and your own wisdom and self-discipline to follow treatment procedures. Take an active part in your treatment, discussing treatment methods and their likely outcome with your therapist and doing whatever you can to optimize their health enhancement. Monitor your own progress and move on when you feel it is necessary or maintain treatment as needed. Even if you don't succeed at first, keep on trying until you find a therapy and therapist that does help you.

The effort you make will be worthwhile for it may bring you not only relief from cystitis but also an improvement in your general health and vitality. You will also have built up a relationship with a reliable practitioner who can help you to stay healthy.

APPENDIX A

# Useful organizations

*This listing is for information only and does not imply any endorsement, nor do the organizations listed necessarily agree with the views expressed in this book.*

## INTERNATIONAL

**International Federation of Practitioners of Natural Therapeutics**
10 Copse Close
Sheet
Petersfield
Hampshire GU31 4DL, UK
Tel 01730 266790
Fax 01730 260058

## AUSTRALASIA

**Acupuncture Ethics and Standards Organization**
PO Box 84
Merrylands
New South Wales 2160
Australia

**Australian Natural Therapists Association**
PO Box 308
Melrose Park
South Australia 5039
Tel 618 297 9533
Fax 618 297 0003

**Australian Traditional Medicine Society**
PO Box 442 or
Suite 3, First Floor,
120 Blaxland Road
Ryde
New South Wales 2112
Tel 612 808 2825
Fax 612 809 7570

**International Federation of Aromatherapists**
35 Bydown Street
Neutral Bay
New South Wales 2089
Australia

**New Zealand Natural Health Practitioners Accreditation Board**
PO Box 37–491
Auckland
Tel 9 625 9966

**New Zealand Register of Acupuncturists**
PO Box 9950
Wellington 1

**NORTH AMERICA**

**Allergy Information Association**
25 Poynter Drive, Suite 7
Weston
Ontario
Tel 718 624 6495

**American Academy of Medical Preventics**
6151 West Century Boulevard
Suite 1114
Los Angeles
California 90045
Tel 213 645 5350

**American Aromatherapy Association**
PO Box 3609
Culver City
California 90231

**American Association of Acupuncture and Oriental Medicine**
National Acupuncture Headquarters
1424 16th Street NW
Suite 501
Washington DC 300 36

**American Association of Naturopathic Physicians**
2800 East Madison Street
Suite 200
Seattle
Washington 98112
*or*
PO Box 20386
Seattle
Washington 98102
Tel 206 323 7610
Fax 206 323 7612

**American Holistic Medical Association**
4101 Lake Boone Trail
Suite 201
Raleigh
North Carolina 27607
Tel 919 787 5146
Fax 919 787 4916

**Bladder Health Council**
300 West Pratt Street
Suite 401
Baltimore MD 21201

**Canadian Holistic Medical Association**
700 Bay Street
PO Box 101, Suite 604
Toronto
Ontario M5G 1Z6
Tel 416 599 0447

**Interstitial Cystitis Foundation**
PO Box 1553
Madison Square Station
New York
NY 10159

**North American Society of Homeopaths**
4712 Aldrich Avenue
Minneapolis 55409

**The Simon Foundation for Continence**
PO Box 835
Wilmette, IL 60091

**SOUTHERN AFRICA**

**Food Allergy and Intolerance Society**
PO Box 22184
Glenashley 4022

**South African Homeopaths, Chiropractors and Allied Professions Board**
PO Box 17055
0027 Groenkloof
Transvaal
Tel 27 1246 6455

**UK**

**Angela Kilmartin**
75 Mortimer Road
London N1 5AR

**British Nutrition Foundation**
15 Belgrave Square
London SW1X 8PS

**National Action on Incontinence**
4 St Pancras Way
London NW1 0PE

**National Society for Research into Allergy**
PO Box 45
Hinckley
Leics. LE10 1JY

**Women's Nutritional Advisory Service**
PO Box 268
Lewes
East Sussex BN7 2QN

**British Allergy Foundation**
St Bartholomews Hospital
West Smithfield
London EC1A 7BE
Tel 0171 600 6127

**British Association for Counselling**
1 Regent Place
Rugby
Warwicks CV21 2PJ
Tel 01788 578328/9

**British Association of Psychotherapists**
37 Mapesbury Road
London NW2 4HJ
Tel 0181 452 9823
Fax 0181 452 5182

**British Complementary Medicine Association**
39 Pretsbury Road
Pitville
Cheltenham
Gloucestershire GL52 2PT
Tel 01242 226770
Fax 01242 226778

**British Holistic Medical Association**
Trust House
Royal Shrewsbury Hospital
South Shrewsbury
Shropshire SY3 8XF
Tel 01743 261155
Fax 01743 3536373

**British Homeopathic Association**
27a Devonshire Street
London W1N 1RJ

**British Medical Acupuncture Association**
Newton House
Newton Lane
Lower Whitley
Warrington
Cheshire WA4 4JA
Tel 01925 730727

**British Society for Allergy and Clinical Immunology**
55 New Cavendish Street
London W1M 7RE
Tel 0171 486 0531

**British Society for Nutritional Medicine**
Stone House
9 Weymouth Street
London W1N 3FF
Tel 0171 436 8532

**Council for Acupuncture**
179 Gloucester Place
London NW1 6DX
Tel 0171 724 5756

**Council for Complementary & Alternative Medicine**
179 Gloucester Place
London NW1 6DX
Tel 0171 724 9103
Fax 0171 724 5330

**Health Education Authority**
Hamilton House
Mabledon Place
London WC1H 9TX
Tel 0171 383 3833
Fax 0171 387 0550

**Institute for Complementary Medicine**
PO Box 194
London SE16 1QZ
Tel 0171 237 5165
Fax 0171 237 5175

**Kanpo Association (Japanese Herbal Practitioners)**
31 Bankhurst Road
London SE6 4XN
Tel 0181 314 1738

**National Institute of Medical Herbalists**
56 Longbrook Street
Exeter
Devon EX4 6AH
Tel 01392 426022
Fax 01392 498963

**Register of Chinese Herbal Medicine**
PO Box 400
Wembley
Middlesex HA9 9NZ
Tel 0181 904 1357

**Society of Teachers of the Alexander Technique (STAT)**
20 London House
266 Fulham Road
London SW10 9EL
Tel 0171 351 0828

**Yoga Biomedical Trust**
PO Box 140
Cambridge CB4 3SY
Tel 01223 67301

**Yoga for Health Foundation**
Ickwell Bury
Biggleswade
Bedfordshire SG18 9EF
Tel 01767 627271

APPENDIX B

# Useful further reading

*A Guide to Acupuncture*, Peter Firebrace and Sandra Hill (Constable, UK, 1994)

*Acupressure for Health*, Jacqueline Young (Thorsons, UK/HarperCollins, USA, 1993)

*Clinical Ecology*, Dr George Lewith and Dr Julian Kenyon (Thorsons, UK, 1985)

*Conquering Cystitis*, Dr Patrick Kingsley (Ebury Press, UK, 1987)

*Coping Successfully with Your Irritable Bladder*, Dr Jennifer Hunt (Sheldon Press, UK, 1995)

*Cystitis, How to prevent infection and inflammation*, Angela Kilmartin (Thorsons, UK, 1994)

*Diets to Help Cystitis*, Ralph McCutcheon (Thorsons, UK, 1980)

*Eating and Allergies*, Robert Eagle (Futura, UK, 1982)

*Food Combining for Health*, Doris Grant and Jean Joice (Thorsons, UK, 1984)

*Natural Fertility Awareness*, John and Farida Davidson (C W Daniel, UK, 1988)

*Nutritional Medicine*, Dr Stephen Davies and Dr Alan Stewart (Pan, UK, 1987)

*Nutritional Therapy*, Linda Lazarides (Thorsons, UK/USA 1996)

*Self-Massage*, Jacqueline Young (Thorsons, UK/HarperCollins, USA, 1992)

*The Essential Book of Herbal Medicine*, Simon Mills (Arkana, UK, 1991)

*The Art of Reflexology*, Inge Dougans and Suzanne Ellis (Element Books, UK, 1992)

*The Complete Family Guide to Alternative Medicine* (Element Books, UK, 1996)

*The Encyclopaedia of Essential Oils*, Julia Lawless (Element Books, UK, 1992)

*The Encyclopaedia of Flower Remedies*, Clare Harvey and Amanda Cochrane (Thorsons, UK, 1995)

*The Family Guide to Homoeopathy*, Andrew Lockie (Hamish Hamilton, UK, 1990)

*The New Holistic Herbal*, David Hoffman (Element Books, UK, 1996)
*Yoga for Common Ailments*, Robert Munroe (Gaia Books, UK, 1994)
*You Are What You Eat*, Kirsten Hartvig and Nic Rowley (Piatkus, UK, 1996)
*You Can Heal Your Life*, Louise Hay (Eden Grove, USA, 1988)

# Index

acidic 2, 8, 17, 100–101
acupressure 26, 34, 51, 57–9
acupuncture x, 16, 27, 47, 48, 50, 51, 53–7
affirmations 90–1
Alexander Technique 29, 51, 58–61
alkaline 17, 28, 100
alkalizing agent 32, 33, 39, 40
allergies 2, 12, 17, 28, 51, 65–70
Angela Kilmartin's bottle-washing 21, 22, 33
antibiotics 19, 29, 30, 36, 39, 40, 41, 44, 65
anti-*candida* diet 35, 68
anti-fungals 41, 67
anxiety x, 19, 30, 90, 94, 99
aromatherapy 34, 51, 61–4

babies 14, 22, 26
bacteria 12, 14, 15
Bach flower remedies 32, 34, 96, 97
balance 46, 61, 66, 82, 86
*Bifidobacterium bifidus* 30, 67
bladder ix, 1, 5, 6, 8, 15–16, 24–5, 26, 34, 42, 53, 58, 60, 86, 90
bottle-washing procedure 21, 22

camomile tea 32, 34
*candida* ix, 19, 24, 35, 41, 65, 67–9
  anti-*candida* diet 68
  symptoms of 67
CAT scan 43
causes 2, 11ff, 46
*chi kung* 25
childbirth 15, 86, 87
children 4, 14, 16, 22, 26
Chinese herbs 76–8
chiropractic 51, 85–8
cleansing fasts 24
clinical ecology 51, 65–70
cognitive therapy 51, 90
congenital (weakness) 16, 26
constipation 15, 24
contraception (forms of) 13, 16–17, 27
counselling 30, 51
  and psychotherapy 93–5, 99
cranberry juice 34, 74–6, 83, 85
cranial osteopathy 58, 86
Cystitis First Aid Kit 31–2

dehydration 12, 18
diagnosis 9, 11, 54
diet 2, 11, 17, 24, 28, 51, 66–7, 68, 83, 87
  and nutrition 51, 100
digestion 15, 24
diuretics 18, 34
douche(s) 17, 21, 23, 28, 63
drug(s) 9, 40–2

elimination diet (for allergy testing) 66–7
emergency self-help 31–3, 37
emotional (aspect) x, 31, 47
emotions 90
endorphins 55, 92
environment 18, 29, 46
  (al) agents 65
episiotomy 16
*Escherichia coli* (*E. coli*) 12, 15, 38

fasts, cleansing 24
fasting 35, 83
First Aid procedure 31, 33
flower remedies 34, 51, 96, 97
fluid intake, inadequate/excess 12
food additives, colourings 17, 28
  allergies 69
  intolerances ix
  irritants 12

general health 46, 53, 55, 60

healing 50, 51, 70–72
healthy diet 34, 100–2
herbal medicine x, 33, 34, 48, 50, 51, 55, 72–8
holistic approach 45
homeopathy x, 34, 50, 51, 78–81
hydrotherapy and physiotherapy 84
hygiene (good/poor) ix, 12, 13–14, 21, 23, 24, 55, 87, 88
hypnotherapy 48, 51, 96, 98

impaired immune function 15
inflammation 1, 2, 8, 12, 14, 15
interstitial cystitis 13
irritants 14, 17, 27, 28

Jacobson's Progressive Relaxation 98

Kanpo (Japanese herbal medicine) 73, 78
kidneys ix, 5, 16–17, 25, 26, 42, 53, 58, 60, 86, 90

*Lactobacillus acidophilus* 30, 67
lifestyle 2, 11, 12, 77, 87
linseed 24
liquid intake 17, 18
  fast 83
lymph 15, 18, 28, 29, 53, 86

manipulative therapies 85–8
massage 51, 55, 64, 82, 88
medication 19, 29, 40
meditation 51, 98
mental affirmation 35
mental aspect x, 47
  image 48
meridian(s) 54
  exercises 26
  lines 57, 91
microscopy 37
mid-stream urine sample (MSU) 33, 35–6, 37–8
mind, treating the 90ff
mineral: *see* vitamin and mineral balance
Mist Pot Cit 33, 39

natural diuretics 34,
therapies x, 44, 45, 46–7
therapists 103–10
naturopathy 51, 63, 82–5
nephritis 10
nutritional therapy 51
supplements 28, 101–2

Oriental medicine 16, 53, 54, 73
osteopathy 29, 47, 51, 85–8

pelvic floor exercises 24–6
physical therapies 53
positive thinking 91–2
pregnancy 15
posture 18, 28, 29, 58, 60, 86
*probiotics* 30, 67, 85
prostate 4, 6
psychology 94–5
(ical) 30, 47, 90
psychotherapy 51, 94
preventive techniques ix

reflexology 27, 51, 88–9
re-infection ix, 9, 35, 36, 41
relaxation training 51, 98–9
remedies, homoeopathic 79–81
Rescue Remedy (Bach flower) 32, 34, 97

scar tissue 9, 15, 47, 55, 86
self-help x, 21ff, 31, 45
sensitivity plates 39
sex 14, 23
sexual therapy 30, 51, 99
Shiatsu 27, 58, 82
side-effects (of drugs) 41–2
sitz bath 34, 63, 84
smoking 19
sodium/potassium balance 5, 17, 39
stress 19, 30, 63, 90, 98
support groups 31
symptoms 2–3, 9, 12, 46, 50, 65, 66–7, 79–81, 96

tension (and anxiety) 19, 98–9
thrush ix, 15, 19, 30, 35, 41, 44, 65, 70, 75, 85
toilet training 16, 21, 26

urine sample 9, 11, 35–6, 37
test 30, 36, 37–8
urinary function 26, 48, 55, 61, 76, 89
system 1, 5, 7, 47, 57, 89

vaginal douches 17, 28
health 15, 23
infections 24
swabs 10, 41
vitamin and mineral balance 17, 102
visualization 92–3

Western medicine 45, 72
herbalists 73

yoga 25, 26